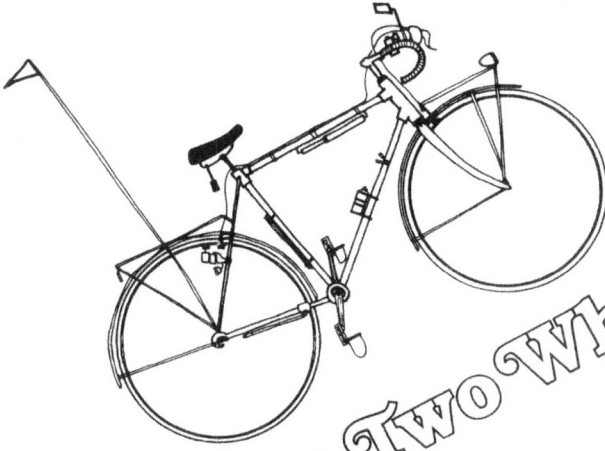

Living on Two Wheels

2nd Edition

Living on Two Wheels

The Complete Guide to Buying, Commuting and Touring

2nd Edition

by Dennis L. Coello

Illustrated by Dennis Nieweg

ROSS BOOKS
Berkeley

Library of Congress Cataloging in Publication Data:
Coello, Dennis.
 Living on Two Wheels
Bibliography: p.
 Includes index
 1. Cycling. 2. Bicycle Touring. 3. Bicycle Commuting. 4. Bicycles. I.
Title.
GV1041.C66 629.2'272 81-10725
ISBN 978-0-89496-061-1 (pbk.)
ISBN 978-0-89496-050-5 (eBook)

Book design by Joan Rhine

Acknowledgements:
Many thanks to Mary Perkins for the tire-removal and tool display drawings. And to David Singer, Gary Topping, and Robert Welsh for their photography assistance. My good friends Doug Conners and Wally Doods read through the first draft and gave suggestions for improvement. Finally, although my wife willingly proof-read the manuscript, I should like to break with tradition by assuring the reader that she, alas, did not type it. That chore fell to me, while she was (in her own words) "too busy making a living."

Publishers Comment:
The first edition of Living on Two Wheels was written some time ago but the concept is just as alive and relevant today as when it was originally written. In this second edition we left the text of the book as it was originally written so the price of a tool, for example, may seem out of date. As far as recources in the indexes are concerned, we updated them and deleted the ones that no longer exist. When looking for equipment we encourage you to do what most people do and simply search the internet using the name of the product you want because we always have some businesses dying and other new ones starting up.

Franz Ross
Fall 2010

This book is dedicated to:

My grandfather, Lyman E. Price, whose infectious love of the outdoors and spirit for adventure have opened worlds for many -

And to my wife, who has shared the long last mile of every ride.

"Oh, come on. You mean to say you don't own a car?"

"That's right."

The look I had grown to expect when I answered this question came upon his face now - a quizzical, half-believing smile.

Then the eyes brightened.

"Get it. Your wife has a car!"

"No," I answered, "she doesn't have one either. As I said, we both get around by bicycle."

The eyes looked down again, perplexed.

"To work and back?"

"Uh-huh."

"And shopping?"

"Yes."

"Winters, too?"

"Sure."

I waited for the usual question - the inevitable next question. It came.

"But how do you do it?"

This book is the answer to that question. Simply, it is the story of five years spent on two wheels. I have tried to record this experience in a manner by which the person fed up with gas lines and gas prices and the hundreds of general motorist hassles can see a way clear of it all. Read on, and you will see why this experiment in simple living without an automobile became, for us, a permanent way of life.

The next few hundred pages can serve as a guide for this transition, or merely as a means of getting the most out of your time on two wheels. You will learn how to shop intelligently for the bicycle best suited to your needs, what kind of frame and group of components to buy, and all the additions to the average bike which I've found necessary for commuting and touring. How to protect yourself while riding in the city, simple maintenance to keep your machine in order, clothing and foul weather gear, saddle-bags and bike carts, ice and snow-riding techniques - it is all here for two hours' reading.

Sixteen years ago I straddled my Raleigh three-speed and headed off on a long journey to Canada and back. Now, many miles and a round-the-world ride later, I h ave to chuckle at how unprepared I was. In short, I tried to write the book I wish I had read before I pedalled my first mile.

D. *Coello*

Foreword

Please don't get the wrong impression. This book is not a polemic against automobiles, nor a fanatical social plan designed to usher in a new world order. The author does not pedal about in Earth Shoes chanting anti-motorist mantras. In fact, I hold a chauffeur's license, and have owned four automobiles during my thirty-odd years of life. For six months I worked in a Dodge dealership tuning up cars, and still own a timing light and dwell-tachometer. In short, I have shared in the American love affair with automobiles. That is, until five years ago, when my wife and I decided to try urban life without a car.

I wish I could claim a heightened degree of social awareness as the primary reason behind my car-less present. We all know, and on most days can see, what the exhausts of thousands of autos do to the air. For that matter automobiles kill 50,000 of us each year, and injure another two million, 150,000 of these permanently (National Safety Council statistics). One of every three of us has been injured by a car.

Nor was patriotism the first impetus to sell my automobile. From the embargo of '73 to the disastrous 1979 oil price hikes, to the hostage crisis of 1980, America has been caught between a terrible dependence upon OPEC petroleum, and a desire to determine freely her foreign policy in the Middle East.

But the real reason behind turning away from cars was not environmental, patriotic, or romantic at all. It was instead a hard-headed, rational, ultimately capitalistic decision. Simply, the profit was gone from the product. Owning and operating a car had become too costly.

The most recent figures on driving an automobile in America are so frightening that few people believe them at first glance. However, the simple but painful process of adding up all the costs - initial purchase price, sales tax, insurance, repairs, license fees, parking, gas and oil, depreciation - of a sub-compact today results in a staggering 38 cents per driven mile. (Hertz Corporation, computing these statistics annually, uses a Pinto as their sub-compact.) Think of it. If you drove ten miles to buy groceries today you've added nearly four dollars to the cost of your food. In larger terms, the average American driver puts ten thousand miles on his car per year. At 38 cents a mile that comes to nearly $4,000. And if you own a car the size of an LTD, the cost jumps another grand, at 48.1 cents per mile.

Perhaps this amount doesn't bother you. You winced the first time you paid a dollar for a gallon of gas, but that was a year ago and now you're used to it. Well, it may soon become much more difficult to roll with the punches. Shell Oil officials have warned of two dollar a gallon gasoline in the very near future. Operating costs have risen 27% in the last year alone. It is as expensive today to run a sub-compact as it was eight years ago to drive a luxury sedan. And, of course, as bad as these figures are, the situation may become one of such limited supply that gas will not be available at any price.

Compare all this to the bicycle. Unlike mass transit it is ready and waiting when you are. Instead of the $5,000 sticker price of a new car, $500 will buy you a lifetime bike and all the commuting gear and tools necessary to care for you and it in the elements. Add to that the cost of this book to teach you how to do it, and you're set.

One final point. Most of us have jobs which fail to keep us in shape, and driving to work is little exercise for anything but an ulcer. Few people have the perseverance to jog or work out regularly, and so we look to the weekends for health. But exercise cannot be infrequent if it is to be good for us. To paraphrase a British physician's report on the subject, exercise must be moderate, regular, continued throughout life, and sufficiently vigorous to bring on slight breathlessness. Commuting to work by bicycle satisfies all these requirements. It is a realistic alternative to the early morning before-work jog we sleep through, and the evening after-work jog we are too tired for.

Exercise, energy, the environment, and cost - all good reasons for switching to two wheels. But let me explain this another way - by recording the experience of mat first year mat my wife, Bopsy, and I turned to bikes.

Five years ago I taught at a school in St. Louis fifteen miles from our apartment. That thirty mile round-trip each day cost me one and a half hours cycling time. My motorist buddies used to kid me about this 'waste' of almost eight hours per week, until I worked out the following defense.

First, I compared the real difference in travel time. I drove to work and home in my aunt's car and found that a thirty mile per hour city speed limit, when combined with traffic, ate up roughly twenty-five minutes each way. Now the 'waste' of time had been cut to forty

cycling time 90 minutes
- driving time 50 minutes
= 40 minute difference

Next, I worked out the difference in transportation expense. (We will use today's figures for both sides of the equation.) The per mile cost is difficult to compute for cycling, as the commuting bicycle requires, on an annual basis, only new tires and tubes, roughly two ounces of oil, one eight ounce tube of grease for the bearings, and two brake pads. Add to this a total investment cost requirement of approximately $500 for the bicycle, tools, bike bag, lock and rain gear, to be stretched over several decades. Next comes fuel cost. Fifteen miles on a bike burns up about six hundred calories, which equals the breakfast of three hotcakes and a glass of milk you would eat even if you drove to work. All this makes it nearly impossible to estimate a per mile expense for bikes, so I will use the figure which one state government has agreed to pay an employee who used his bike on the job - 4 cents. Using the figures of 38 cents per mile for a sub-compact, and 4 cents per mile for a bike, the difference in daily travel cost comes to $10.20. Over a school year of one hundred-eighty days I had therefore saved, or paid myself for cycling $1,836!

Car

30 miles per day
x 38 cents per mile
$11.40 cost per day

Bike

30 miles per day
x 4 cents per mile
$1.20 cost per day

$11.40
-1.20
$10.20 difference

Annual savings: 180 days x $10.20 = $1,836.

But this isn't the total picture. Consider the fact that if I hadn't been pedalling thirty miles a day, and if I wished to remain in shape. I'd have had to work out five days a week. The most similar exercise would have been Jogging, with the roughly equivalent distance of three miles requiring eighteen to twenty minutes of actual running, and at least ten minutes for dressing before and showering afterward. Now our computations stand as follows.

Car
$11.40 cost per day
50 minute travel time
+ 30 minute exercise
$11.40, 80 minutes

Bike
$1.29 cost per day
+ 90 minute travel time
$1.20, 90 minutes

Simply, saving ten minutes daily would have cost me $10 a day. By this point, feeling my defense of commuting by bike iron-clad, my friends would begin arguing the convenience angle of car-ownership. And here they had me. My lifestyle was more problematical, as it conflicted with a world of automobiles. I had to rent a car on occasion, or forgo a late dinner invitation on the other side of town. Yet I was sure that in time these problems would disappear, that a world awakened to the need for conservation of natural resources would re-orient its cities accordingly, that customs would change to incorporate the slower-paced, less frenetic future. That was 1975. Now, five years later, such changes are becoming evident. 'Nucleus' cities of 100,000 people are being planned, where jobs, stores, houses and entertainment will all be geographically proximate. The ever-increasing cost of gasoline is making people think twice before buying homes far from work, and greatly decreasing 'impulsive' driving. Time tests conducted in New York and Washington, D.C., have shown bicycles actually beating cars in cross-town travel. And, finally, what is most encouraging of all, people whom I never expected to take the plunge have asked me about commuting by bike. Things are looking up.

Contents

Part One
The Purchase

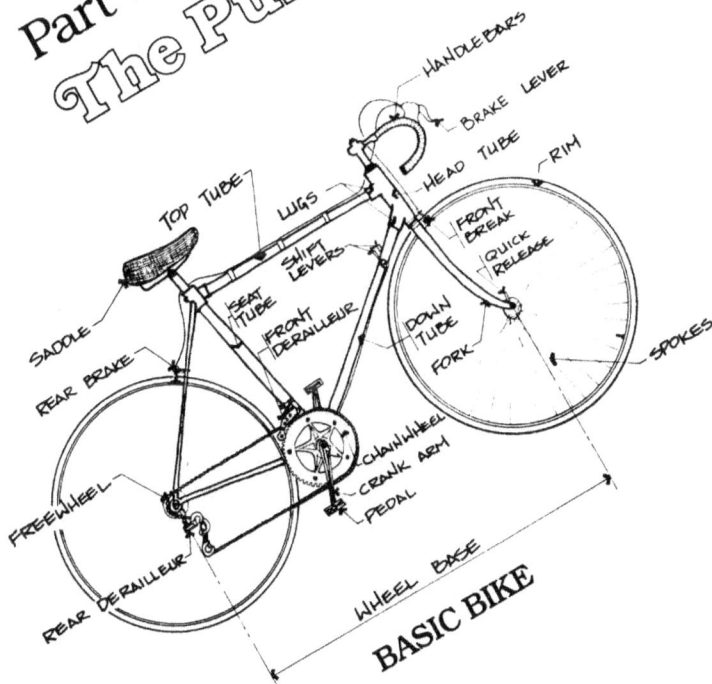

HANDLEBARS

BRAKE LEVER

HEAD TUBE

RIM

TOP TUBE

LUGS

FRONT BREAK

QUICK RELEASE

SHIFT LEVER

SEAT TUBE

FRONT DERAILLEUR

DOWN TUBE

FORK

SADDLE

SPOKES

REAR BRAKE

CHAINWHEEL

CRANK ARM

PEDAL

FREEWHEEL

REAR DERAILLEUR

WHEEL BASE

BASIC BIKE

1. Buying the Right Bike

Chances are when you decide to begin commuting by bicycle and leave the car in the garage, or sell the thing completely and prepare for the new decade by heading to the bike shop, the very look of the new breed of two-wheeled mounts will scare you. What happened to that sturdy-looking frame and those big tires? Where did the old handlebars go, and the big cushioned seat with springs in the bottom? And your coaster brakes applied by pedalling backward - now it's to be done by hand? But don't be put off. Every change was made for a reason, and you as the rider will benefit from it once the initial shock has subsided.

One warning. Don't back away when this first part becomes difficult. One of the nicest things of all about cycling is that in time every rider can maintain his machine, and with only a modest outlay of cash for tools.

The salesman in the bike shop has just looked up from his order book to see you standing in front of him. You are smiling. He is not. He is the first bike salesman you've seen today, but he's seen ten other customers in the last two hours who began with the same smile and the same sentence, "Uh, I want to buy a bike..." He turns from you and approaches a rack of machines across the shop floor.

"This one." he begins in a dull, uninterested monotone, "is a Fuji S-12-S. Lugged frame, double-butted, cotterless crank, quick-release wheels front and rear. About $380."

Lugged? Double-butted? Cotterless crank? Quick release? So you thought this would all be kid-stuff, eh? Sorry to disappoint you, but it's an increasingly sophisticated world. When Bopsy and I made the switch from cars we were fortunate in already knowing the rudiments of frames and components. But in case the salesman's words are Greek to you, the following pages should be helpful. I promised this would be a simple guide, and it will be. Just stay with me and refer to the pictures to keep things clear.

Lugs

Look at the bike the salesman has in his hands. The frame is really a combination of tubes - one that runs from just below the saddle to the handlebars (top tube), another from the saddle straight down to the pedals (seat tube), a third from the pedals to the headset (down tube). Sort of a triangle. Attached to this are the tubes extending to the rear (chain and seat stays). Okay, how are these tubes held together? One way is to braze or weld them in place. But this isn't the strongest method, unless the joints are mitered (fitted together at precise angles) with great care, and at considerable cost. A lugged frame uses lugs to hold the tubes in place - metal joints which fit around the tubes like a sleeve and thus add their own strength to that of the original welded bonding. Now don't get confused. Just remember that a good bike in the medium price range ($250 - $400) should be lugged, and will be stronger for it.

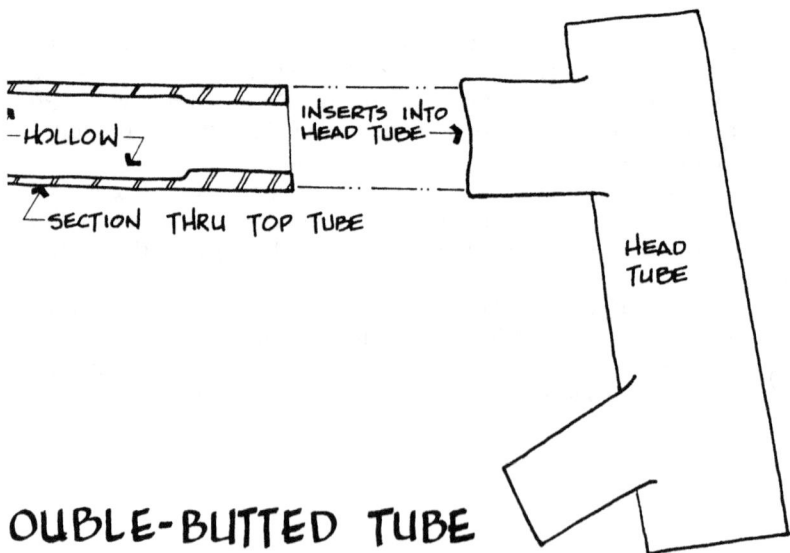

HOLLOW

SECTION THRU TOP TUBE

INSERTS INTO HEAD TUBE →

HEAD TUBE

OUBLE-BUTTED TUBE

Double-butted

The second thing the salesman said in his description of the bike was "double-butted." Whereas I have heard this term used to describe the rear-view of a large rider on a narrow saddle, in the bike shop it refers to the frame. The tubes of a frame are hollow, and in the old days the thickness of the tube walls was the same throughout (straight-gauge tubing). But if the bike is double-butted, the tube wall is thinnest at the middle, and thickest at both ends where it joins the other tubes. (A 'butted' tube is thicker at only one end.) The reason for this is that the greatest points of stress are at the ends of the tube near the joints, and thus a reinforcement here adds strength where it is needed. A second reason is that where the strength is not needed - in the middle - the tube can remain thin and thus light in weight. All this takes place inside the tube, by the way. You won't see any difference on the outside tube measurements. (It's interesting that this idea supposedly came from 'human engineering' - our bones are double-butted as well.)

Fork-rake, Wheel base

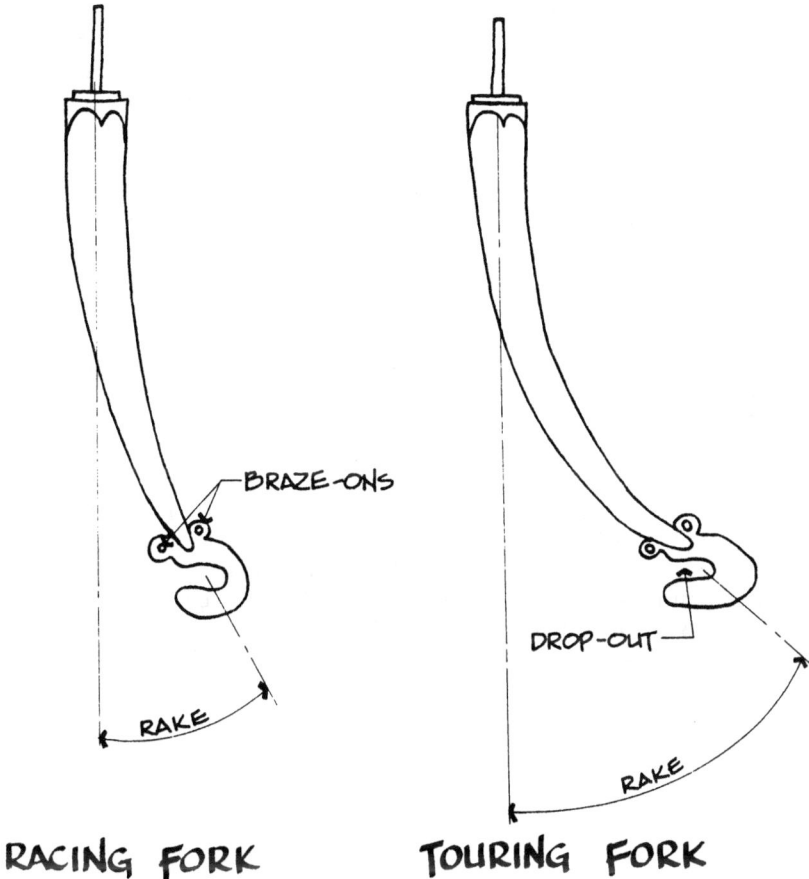

RACING FORK   TOURING FORK

Another point to discuss with the salesman is something called 'fork-rake'. This is a measurement of the angle of the fork from where it leaves the head tube to where it attaches to the front wheel axle. If the fork-rake angle is small then the fork will look pretty straight to you, and the front and rear wheels will be close together. If the fork-rake angle is great, the fork will have quite a curve to it, and therefore the front and rear wheels will be further apart. This last measurement, the distance between the front and rear wheels, is called the 'wheel base' - measured from front axle to rear axle. The shorter the wheel base (small rake angle, straight fork), the stiffer the ride. Racing bikes are built this way - quick, responsive, with every bump in the road transmitted to the rider. The longer the wheel base (greater rake angle, more curved fork), the softer the ride. Touring bikes are built in this manner. Ask about the wheel base; compare the forks of several machines. And think about the kind of riding you'll be doing. I use my one bike for every mile I pedal, and find the longer wheel base both comfortable cross-country and sufficiently responsive for commuting in town.

Frame composition

Now that you know the overall design of a frame, we must deal with the question of frame material - the metal with which the tubes, forks and stays are made. There are three elements in the discussion:weight, strength, and cost. The first two elements - light weight and great strength cannot be purchased together without considerable expense. Most Americans still think in terms of the forty pound clunkers with balloon tires which they pedalled as kids. Those frames were nearly indestructible, but the strength and relatively low cost came as a result of the poor grade heavy-weight piping used for tubes. Conversely, several years ago I saw an inexpensive light-weight ten speed bike which had a broken top tube - head tube connection. In this case a poor grade light-weight frame without lugs had broken under stress. Therefore, realize that an investment in a good quality, light frame will literally last you a lifetime, and provide dependable and enjoyable service along the way.

There is a good chance that when you walk into the bike shop you'll find two or more of the following frame brands: Vitus, Reynolds, Tange, Columbus, and Ishiwata. On some you'll see numbers like 1020, 022, and 531. If you ask about them the informed reply will contain words like 'ferrous steel alloys', 'chrome-moly', manganese-molybdenum, and 'high carbon tubing'. A bike shop owner who really knows his product, like Tom McKnight of Salt Lake and Bill Logan of St. Louis, might explain that with Reynolds tubing the number 531 at one time referred to the ratio of manganese, molybdenum, and carbon in the frame material. He might go on to say that Columbus frames are chrome molybdenum, that they are a bit stiffer in their ride, and therefore are preferred by racers. If the shop isn't busy he might continue with an explanation of how seamless tubing is formed, and a fascinating description of the geometry of frame angles. And, at the end of an hour, when he is satisfied that you now are fully informed of the chemical balance in all bike metals, you will look at him sheepishly and ask, "But, which is the best?"

Let me try to make it clearer for you. What you want is a bike which weighs in around twenty-eight pounds or less, and is made with seamless tubing. (If you're in a good bike shop you won't find seamed tubing even if you look for it - it's usually used for department store junkers.) If you can afford it, the Reynolds 531 can't be beaten for light weight, strength, and quality. But, if you can't go Reynolds, or the equally expensive Columbus, don't despair. You probably won't detect difference between those frames and the steel alloys.

Frame styles

Most of us remember the old classifications - the man's bike had the bar across the top and the woman's bike didn't. Well, you can still buy a woman's bike. But please don't.

Imagine holding a small triangle in your hands, three pieces of metal soldered together. Now, holding two sides of this triangle in your fingertips, try to bend it. Depending upon the metal and the quality of the soldering job you probably won't find this easy to do. However, imagine now that one of the three sides of this small triangle is gone, that in your hands you now hold merely two pieces attached at one end - a V rather than a triangle. Try to bend it. Of course, you'll find it considerably easier.

This simple experiment should make it clear why the 'ladies' model is unacceptable for commuting and touring. A third frame style is now on the market, however, which combines the strength of the men's with the ease of getting on and off the ladies' bike, and allows her to ride in a skirt. This is the 'mixte', which, like the men's model, gains its strength from a bar running from the headset to the seat tube - but angling downward from the headset to meet the seat tube just above the bottom bracket. This closes the V of the down tube and seat tube, yet still leaves room to step through the frame. My choice is still the men's model for touring, but a good mixte should give no trouble on the hardest commuting routes, or on tour with light loads.

Cranks

Our salesman used the term "cotterless crank" following his description of the frame. The reference is to the best of three methods of crank attachment, best for reasons which I'll give in a minute. Look at the overall bike diagram again, and you'll see where the crank is. Most of the old single speed coaster bikes had one-piece cranks which included the crankarms (to which the pedals are attached) the bottom bracket axle, and the front sprocket. Of course, with this system you couldn't change the size of the front sprocket to vary your gearing or switch to longer or shorter crankarms without swapping the entire

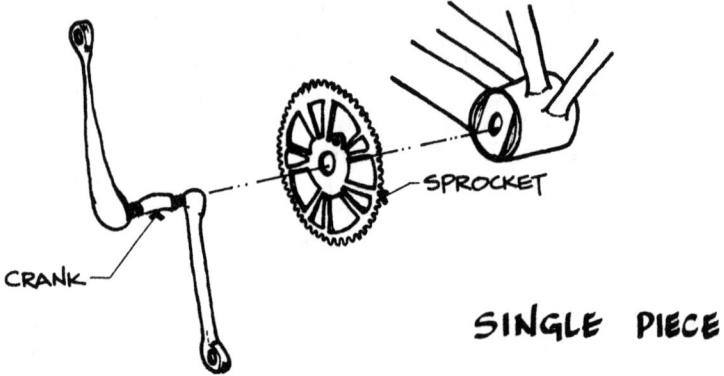

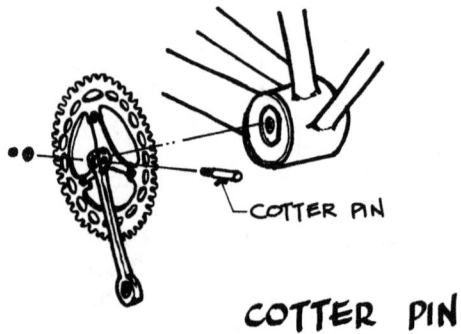

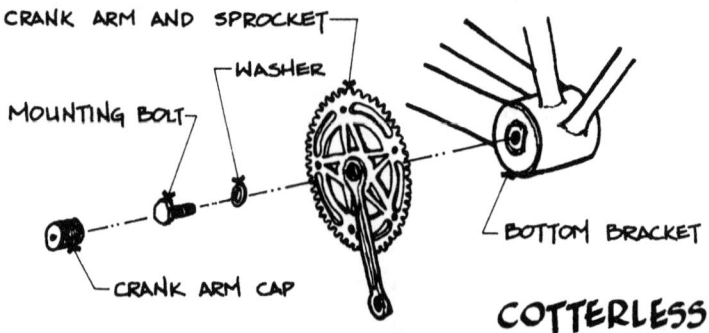

CRANK

SPROCKET

SINGLE PIECE

COTTER PIN

COTTER PIN

CRANK ARM AND SPROCKET

WASHER

MOUNTING BOLT

CRANK ARM CAP

BOTTOM BRACKET

COTTERLESS

set-up. (Very tall riders sometimes prefer longer than standard 170 mm crankarms.) Also, if the teeth of the sprocket wore out after many years of hard use, or if the crankarm threads for the pedal attachment stripped out, the whole apparatus was shot.

An improvement upon this method was the cotter-pin system, which allowed for a separation of the crankarm, sprocket, and bottom bracket axle (also called a 'spindle'). The cotter-pin held the crankarms onto the axle, and had merely to be driven out for removal. But I use the word 'merely' in jest. Anyone who has not had the unfortunate experience of 'removal and replacement' (as the inoffensive phrase goes in mechanics manuals) of the pin cannot begin to appreciate the cotterless system. I once had to drill a hole into the head of the cotter-pin, heat the crankarm with a propane torch, and beat the pin out with a hammer to jar it from its snug home. At every rap I winced at the thought of what effect this might be having upon the ball bearings inside the bottom bracket. You can imagine that one's recourse in such a situation is not to 'remove and replace' the pin at all - which is possible if the rider foregoes the necessary repacking of bottom bracket bearings in fresh grease once a year, and if hard pedalling does not offset the cotter-pin in the middle of a tour.

I recall very clearly the first cotterless crank assembly I owned, for reasons which should now be fairly obvious. With this arrangement a crankarm mounting bolt replaces the cotter-pin in its purpose of affixing the arm to the axle. The latter is threaded to receive the bolt, which passes through the arm and is then covered by a 'dust cap'. Removal is made possible by a crank tool or crank extractor. I will describe this tool's use in the chapter on mechanics.

You know now to purchase a bicycle which has the cotterless system, for frequent maintenance to the bottom bracket preserves the axle and bearings and allows for easy pedalling. But in order to leave the bike shop with the best machine for your money, and one which will give no trouble on the road, we must say more about crankset parts. The front sprockets (also called 'chainrings') are, on most good cranksets, separate from the crankarms. (They are held together by 'chainring fixing bolts' when on the bike.) This provides the rider with opportunity of switching the size of the chainrings depending upon the adversity of the tour ahead of him, or again the ability to replace a worn-out sprocket without also replacing the arm, as necessary with the single-piece crankarm sprocket. The right-hand crankarm (right as you sit on the bike) will have either three or five 'pins'. These pins are really the arms which reach out to the chainrings. Be sure to buy a five-pin crankarm, for it will keep the chainring more in 'true' than the three-pin, thereby relieving you of a host of front derailleur problems which I'll deal with in the mechanics chapter.

Alright, thus far you have a cotterless crank with a five-pin arm. Now the decision is what size chainrings you should buy. Remember that the salesman is not going to pump your bicycle up any hills - *you* are. And therefore chances are he will try to sell whatever 'gearing' ratio is stock for that bicycle line. That may be a 52-48, a 52-46 (number of teeth in large and small chainrings respectively), or almost any combination the manufacturer thought profitable. It will cost a few dollars extra to have some changes made, but the first time you pedal uphill with a load of groceries, or against a strong headwind, you'll appreciate the investment. And now for an explanation of the numbers above, and all this 'gearing' business in general.

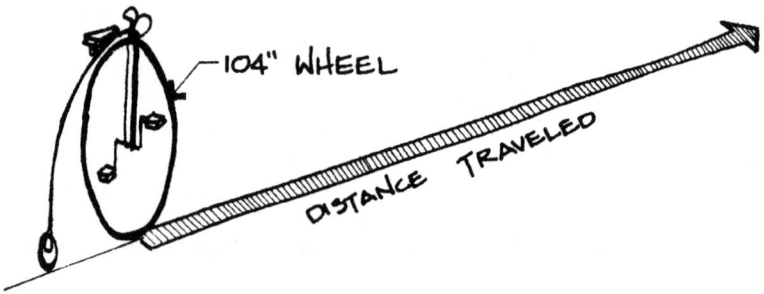

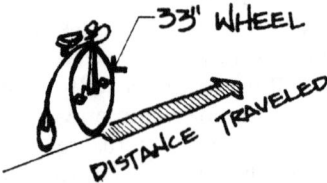

104" WHEEL

DISTANCE TRAVELED

33' WHEEL

DISTANCE TRAVELED

GEAR RATIOS

Gearing

A trip to the bike shop will introduce you to one, three, five, ten, twelve, fifteen, and eighteen 'speed' bicycles. The 'speed' in this refer-ence is to the number of varying gear ratios available. Most of us who are over thirty began with a 'one-speed', a single sprocket or chainring up front, and a single sprocket in the rear (that is, attached to the rear wheel). When we sat on the seat and pedalled once, the rear wheel would go around 1 1/2 or 2 or 3 times, depending upon the difference in size of the front and rear sprockets. Imagine a huge front sprocket and a very tiny rear, and how many times the rear sprocket would be turned by the time you pedalled the chainring around just once. (Even if you are equipped with only the slightest degree of mechanical aptitude you should be able to see how much harder it is to pedal when the size of the chainring is many times that of the small rear sprocket.) Well, the old single speed balloon tire bike was okay for spinning around the neighborhood and jumping curbs, but it wasn't adaptable to differences in terrain. Think of the way you change your stride when walking or hiking - long steps covering maybe three feet at a time on level ground, and short, choppy steps of a foot each when going up a steep hill. If you tried to make those long strides going up hills you'd soon wear yourself out and have to stop.

It's the same way on a bike. If you have a 27" wheel (27" in diameter - standard for most ten-speed bikes sold today) which turns one time with each revolution on the front sprocket, you move yourself down the road almost 85 inches, or 7 feet each time you pedal. (This figure comes by multiplying the diameter of the wheel by pi - 27" x 3.14 = 84.78".) If the rear wheel turns 3 times with each revolution of the pedals you increase your distance travelled to 21 feet. Now, if your single-speed bike is set up with the first of these two gear patterns you'll do fine going uphill, but you won't be able to pedal going downhill at all, and you'll wear yourself out trying to get anywhere on level terrain. If you rode a single-speed bike with a gear pattern making the rear wheel revolve 3 times with each pedal rotation, you'd zoom down the highway on level ground, but have to walk up all but the slightest of hills. Naturally, the next development was to create a bike with several gearing possibilities - and thus came the 3-speed.

My heart always warms a bit when I see a bike that reminds me of my old Raleigh 3-speed, with a red frame and silver fenders and a Sturmey-Archer 'twist-grip' gear changing device. I rode that beautiful bike 1,700 miles on a trip to Canada and back, and had no mechanical problems. However, I recall many times in Canada wishing for a 'lower' gear - easier to pedal, and then there were some good days with the wind at our backs when I wished for a 'higher' gear - harder to pedal and therefore covering more ground with every pump. That's the trouble with 3-speeds; the extremes in gearing are not very far apart, and if any trouble arises the rider must break down the rear hub, which looks like a watch inside. (On a 3-speed all the gearing is housed inside the large rear wheel hub; on other-speed bikes this gearing is all external.) My buddy Roy Longuet and I took our 3-speed hubs apart before the Canada trip, determined to learn every detail before heading out. I remember removing the gear housing cover very carefully, allowing our first peek inside. Our eyes fixed upon a jeweler's paradise of pawl springs and planet gears and cartridge retaining rings. I was sixteen then, my buddy fifteen, and we had never done anything more complicated to our bikes than fix flats and oil the chain. We looked at one another silently, without comment replaced the housing cover, and prayed all summer that we'd have no gear trouble on the road.

A 5-speed bike has a single sprocket up front and a 'cluster' (freewheel) of five sprockets in the rear. By derailing the chain from one to another of these rear sprockets (with the use of a 'derailleur') the rider has five gears available to him. Add a second chainring or sprocket up front and the bike becomes a 10-speed (2 sprockets front x 5 sprockets rear = 10 gears possible); add a sixth sprocket in the rear for a 12-speed (2 front x 6 rear = 12). A third chainring provides a 15-speed, and the addition of a sixth sprocket in the rear increases this to an 18-speed. That is really all you need to know about gearing to understand the differences between the 'speed' bikes, but let me add a little more here to explain the confusing lingo you might have thrown your way in the shop.

Many bike manufacturers will publish literature on their cycles which states something like "33 to 101 gear range as equipped," or "100 inch gear high range." What is a 100 inch gear, and how is that number derived? It comes from this formula.

$$\frac{\text{\# teeth in front sprocket}}{\text{\# teeth in rear sprocket}} \times \text{ wheel diameter in inches}$$

Take my bike for example: the large front sprocket has 54 teeth, the smallest back sprocket has 14.

$$(54/14) \times 27 = 104 \text{ inch gear}$$

But this does not mean the bike will travel 104 inches down the road with one pump of the pedals. If refers instead to the number of inches in diameter the front wheel would be in a 'direct-drive' set up, such as the old 'high-wheelers' during the 1870's and 1880's. Those bikes had no complicated gearing, and therefore the single 'gear' was determined by the size of the front wheel, to which the pedals were attached. Imagine a high-wheeler 104 inches in diameter, or more than 8½ feet high!

On the other end of the scale the lowest gear on my bike is 33.3 inches:

$$(42/34) \times 27 = 33.3$$

In this case the 'high-wheeler' wouldn't be so high at all, and would look more like a child's tricycle. Now you can see the beauty of today's gearing, which provides for such extremes of great speed and hill climbing potential, and all the gradients in between. (A full gear chart may be found in the appendix.)

Years ago, before I knew any better, I bought a bike which had two nearly equal front sprockets. It was still a 10-speed, and to me they were all the same. Don't make that mistake. Be sure your smaller front sprocket is considerably smaller than the larger chainring. My larger chainring is a 54 tooth, my smaller a 42. When combined with a widespread cluster of sprockets in the rear (14, 16, 02, 28, 34), I have all the extremes at either end that I'll want. (On our worlder in '74, however, we did drop to a 38 tooth small chainring, which helped greatly in climbing the Eastern Ghats of India.) Some bikes come standard today with the wide range of gear ratios necessary for touring and easy commuting. Look for these bikes, or pay the few extra dollars to change the front sprockets and freewheel. People who are mechanics first and riders second will argue that such wide ranges cause a duplication of gear ratios. For example, when I am on my smaller chainring and middle sprocket of my freewheel I have a 51.5" gear. When on my larger chainring and fourth largest freewheel sprocket I have a 52" gear. That bothers mechanics. But it doesn't make any difference to the commuter or rider on tour, who is primarily interested in the extreme low and high gears, and good ratios between. Most people will drop to their small chainring only for hard climbs anyway, and use it with just the two or three largest freewheel sprockets. When I commute I use only five gears, shifting only my rear derailleur and staying always in the larger chainring. So don't let the shop mechanic talk you out of a wide gear range potential. Remember that you are doing the pedalling.

Derailleur

This component is the equivalent of your car's transmission. If your bike comes equipped with an inexpensive or low-range derailleur it will not be able to handle the new sizes of sprockets that you request. Don't let that stop you. For only a few dollars more you can purchase a good derailleur which will handle the sprockets, and you'll be riding about in ease. (Sun Tour - the alloy VGT model - is my first choice for low cost and excellent performance. A comparable derailleur which is now showing up on many bikes as standard equipment is the Sun Tour VxGT.)

Shifters

The action of the derailleurs is controlled by the gear shift levers, and here you'll have some choice as to location. Some riders prefer the 'bar-con' shifters, protruding from the handlebar ends. Others like

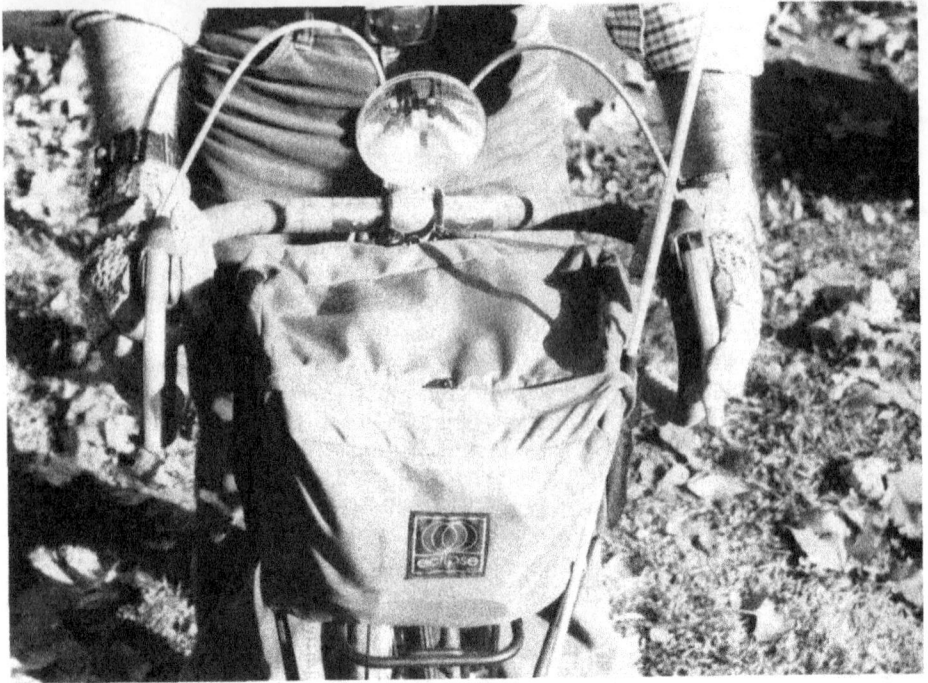

the 'stem' shifters, where the levers are found on either side of the headset or handlebar stem. Personally, I find the latter arrangement awkward to my reach, and the first option disagreeable due to the necessary pressure exerted on the handlebar end when changing gears. My choice is the 'down tube' shifter position, for it is the most convenient of the three. A riders's hand will fall naturally to it when lifted from the bar.

Quick-release

Finally, we come to the last of the terms used by our salesman in the bike shop, a reference to "quick-release" wheels. I will borrow a paragraph from an article on 78 year-old Tullio Campagnalo, who invented the quick-release wheel as a result of the following bicycle race, and went on to develop a line of components unequalled for their meticulous design, excellence in craftsmanship, and high cost.

> In early November of 1927, while he was leading 50 rivals in a 100-mile race through the Dolomites, snow began to fall heavily. Although Campagnalo was wearing only a short-sleeved shirt, he carried on and still held a two-minute lead at the peak altitude of 3,500 feet. Shortly after starting the descent, through 10 inches of snow, he suffered a puncture. While he was trying to get the frozen nuts and lock washers off his wheel to change the tire. several dozen cyclists passed him. [*Sports Illustrated*, Feb. 18, 1980)

Speed of repair is not as crucial in touring, but it is convenient. However, bike thieves also appreciate the convenience of removing a wheel by the mere Hip of the quick-release lever, so lock it up. (See Chapter Three on protecting your investment.) Quick release wheels cost a bit more, but most bikes in the $250 range on up come with them as standard equipment.

I realize it took a long time to explain only the terms lugged, double-butted, cotterless crank, derailleur, shifters, and quick-release. But remember that we went through the entire gearing discussion, which is the most perplexing to beginners. And now for a few more components to know something about when buying or rebuilding your bike.

Handlebars

Handlebars have been changed from the old Texas long-horn style to the 'drop-bars' of today for reasons of control, comfort, and pedalling power. With the old bars there was only one place for your hands if you wanted full control, and that was at the very ends on the handle-grips. The new drop-bars can be held in three positions with good control, which allows for the much needed opportunity of shifting one's posture in the saddle and thus varying the extension of the arms. This has a significant effect upon relieving neck, shoulder, and back muscle tension which results from staying in any one position too long. The last benefit - pedalling power - can be explained through a simple experiment.

Sit upright in a chair with your legs in front of you, feet flat on the floor, and hands held out away from you as if resting upon the old-style handlebar-grips. Now, stand up. You will notice some difficulty doing this; that is, you will find yourself instinctively wanting to draw your feet up under the chair so as to employ the powerful thigh muscles for propulsion. This upright position is the posture which the old-style bars and frame angles required you to assume. Next, sitting again in the chair, but this time with feet drawn up under you, and leaning forward in a bit of a crouch, try to stand. You'll notice the difference immediately, as all your leg muscle is placed where it must be to gain maximum power. This is the 'power' reason for new frame angles and drop-bars, to gain every advantage of leg and upper torso muscle strength.

Perhaps you recall bicycling as exercise only for the legs. If so, cycle ten miles over hilly terrain, and see where you hurt the next day. Forearm and hand muscles will be tired from gripping the bar. Triceps at the back of the arms will feel the effects of near-constant contraction during the ride; biceps, and the pectoralis major and minor chest muscles will be felt from 'pulling' up the hills. (Pulling toward you with the handlebars makes pushing away with the pedals easier.) Inter-costals (rib muscles) will feel the effects of heavy breathing. Back, neck, and shoulders will ache a bit. In short, almost all upper torso muscles are put into play with the new bars and angles. Whereas this won't please you while aching all over, after a week's training you'll begin to see how complementary muscles assist one another to propel you down the road. This not only makes cycling excellent exercise, but makes for an understanding of the almost unbelievable fact that man on a bike is the most efficient animal in the world.

One last thing about handlebars. Some few models still have the 'brake-assist' bars located an inch or so under the regular bar. This was an early attempt, I believe, to get Americans to purchase drop-bars, and escape the complaint about a rider not having his hands close enough to the rakes when riding in a more upright position. Thus some manufacturers resorted to calling this extra weight by the incongruous name of 'safety-bars'. They are surely anything but that. Riders who become accustomed to these additional bars will grab them in an emergency rather than reaching for the hand brakes, and this could be disastrous; safety-bars apply only a portion of real braking power to the wheels, and thus a rider can fail to stop in time. While commuting in heavy traffic I ride with my hands on the brake hoods (or 'hooded brake levers', standard on most bikes today, these are plastic or gum-rubber casings to cushion your palms), ready for quick stops when some motorist cuts me off.

Saddle

If I haven't convinced you that the new drop-bars are a necessary change from the old style I'll never convince you of the need for a switch in the next area - the saddle. Your old balloon tire one-speed had a mattress seat with giant springs on the bottom; your new bike will sport a thin leather saddle only half as wide, with no springs below. At first glance it appears as comfortable as spending a day straddling a fence post. But looks can be deceiving.

Just a word on the old style before discussing which new saddle to buy. One of the problems with the mattress seat was the width which appeared so comforting. After a lot of pedalling, especially in shorts, the insides of a rider's thighs will become chafed from constant contact with the seat. Also, due to springs the seat will never 'form' to the rider, that is, slowly mold to the rider's shape. Finally, some mattress seats have a rough time with the weather. All seats after a few years will have scrapes and tears, usually along the right hand edge from leaning the bike across buildings and fences. On a leather saddle these nicks are no trouble, but on a mattress type the leather or plastic covering when ripped can expose the fabric beneath it to damaging moisture.

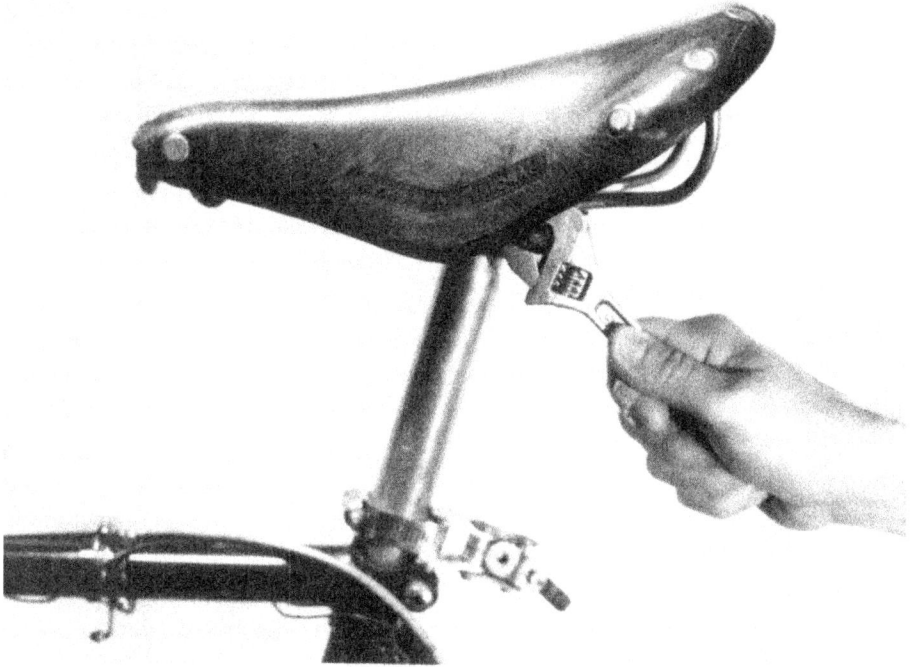

Now you have several reasons for staying away from the mattress seat, and the remaining problem is to choose a good new-style saddle. I have more than 30,000 miles on my Brooks Professional all-leather model, and therefore am partial to it. The Brooks Pro is advertised as a life-time investment, and I do not doubt the claim. But there are some things to know. First, breaking them in is a lengthy and uncomfortable process, though there are ways to hurry this along. Some riders suggest soaking the saddle in neat's foot oil and beating it with a ball bat to soften the leather fibers, but I prefer just to apply the oil on the saddle underside every other day for the first month's riding. (In case you're unfamiliar with this, neat's foot refers to the leather dressing oil produced by boiling the feet and shinbones of a 'neat' - a cow.) Something to watch out for is the dye in the leather which wears off in time, especially when wet. I carry a plastic saddle cover to end the worry of dye stain on my pants in the rain, or after I have saddle-soaped or oiled the leather.

To avoid these problems of a breaking-in period and dye stains, I suggest the Ideale saddle. The natural tan-colored leather will not stain and those Ideales stamped "Daniel Rebour" have received a special conditioning treatment which greatly softens the leather. Generally unavailable in bike shops, you'll have to order the Ideale from the Bikecology catalogue. (Addresses of all catalogues can be found in the Appendix.) Believe me, the comfort is well worth the extra expense.

Another alternative is the Avocet. Two years ago my wife and I took a great ride through the San Juan Islands north of Seattle with several friends. One was riding an Avocet touring saddle, and although it was relatively new, my friend Tom Hansen had no trouble with it. I wrote to the company for information. What came in the return mail was an interesting advertisement - "The Avocet Anatomic Comfort System." The Woman's touring model has a "special anatomical shell to conform with the female pelvic structure." Both male and female models have orthopedic polyurethane padded humps, which are specially molded to give comfort on long hauls. Now, as with wooden skis and bamboo poles in cross-country snow touring, the leather saddle is the way of the purist. However, if this distinction is of little importance to you, and if you demand instant comfort from a saddle, you should test-ride an Avocet.

Brakes

Okay, just a few more items and we'll be out of the bike shop, and onto the road. Most bikes in the $200-$300 price range come with either Weimann or Dia-Compe center-pull brakes. These are fine for a start -or for that matter could do you for a lifetime. My old inexpensive Weimann center-pulls went with me for more than ten years, and I'd still be riding with them if a particular motorist hadn't clobbered me last year and caused me to replace my machine. But a word on the two main types of brakes available. Center-pulls are named that because the braking action comes from the attached top cable being pulled from the center causing the brake pads on either side of the wheel to move together - thus applying pressure on the wheel and slowing its rotation.

Side-pulls are the second main type of brake available. The name again comes from the mechanical action - the brake control cable leading from the handlebars to the brake assembly attaches not at the center but the side. Which kind is preferable? I have ridden many miles with both and find them about equal in all categories except for the lower priced brakes - in the twelve to twenty dollar range. At this price I would go for the center-pull, though the more expensive sets, $25-$80, are primarily side-pull. The brake pads on an inexpensive side-pull will often strike the wheel at different times, giving uneven braking and throwing off one's steering a bit.

Finally, don't forget the 'hoods' over the brake levers.

Pedals

One day in 1966, my buddy and I pulled up in front of a general store in the Texas panhandle. As we dismounted, one old Texan sitting on a wooden bench nearby looked up at us, squinted his eyes a bit in the sun, and said, "Well, I'll be! Stirrups on a bicycle!"

That old gent was referring to the toeclips and straps mounted on our pedals. Most new riders are scared away from toeclips because of a misconception about their purpose. They are not designed to hold your feet firmly to the pedal, or keep you from removing your feet at will. In fact, the Texan made a pretty good comparison with 'Stirrups', for the purpose is nearly the same. Toeclips and straps allow your feet to rest comfortably in place without fear of slipping off. (How many of you when kids had the painful experience of pedalling quickly along on an old balloon tire bike, and suddenly slipping off one pedal and falling onto the top tube?) But an equally important function is the increase of pedal efficiency - by 30% according to some studies.

One of the reasons for this efficiency boost is the fact that with clips and straps the pedals can be propelled in their rotation not only during the 'down-stroke', but assisted on the 'up-stroke' at the same time. I didn't realize this fact until a day in '73 when I tried to ride my bike to college without toeclips. I almost could not ride the four short miles, for on every rotation my foot in the up-stroke position would lift off the pedal - an indication of how much power I usually transmitted through the lifting of the pedals in preparation for the down-stroke.

A second reason for the boost in pedal efficiency with clips and straps is that only the ball of the foot can be placed on the pedal, allowing the foot to act as a powerful fulcrum during rotation. This is accompanied by a technique called 'ankling', which is difficult to learn and tiring at first (proof that it incorporates additional muscles.) However, ankling is often the reason that riders of equal strength pedal at different speeds - the faster rider is exerting no additional energy, but merely making use of the available mechanical energy.

Begin by adjusting your saddle height so that when then pedal is at the end of its down-stroke (6 o'clock) it is too low for your instep or heel to reach it -just the ball of your foot must be on the pedal. At the top of the up-stroke (12 o'clock) the heel should be below the pedal; the foot is actually pointing up slightly at this time, with the heel at about the 11 o'clock position. Now, on the beginning downstroke, not

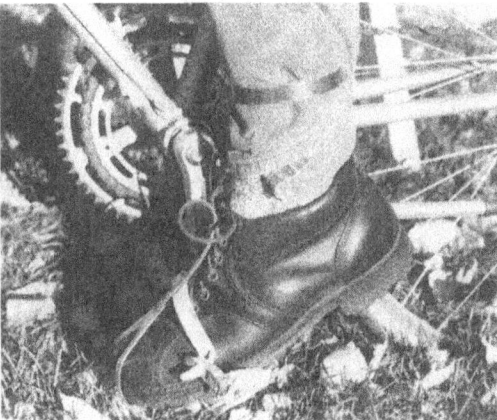

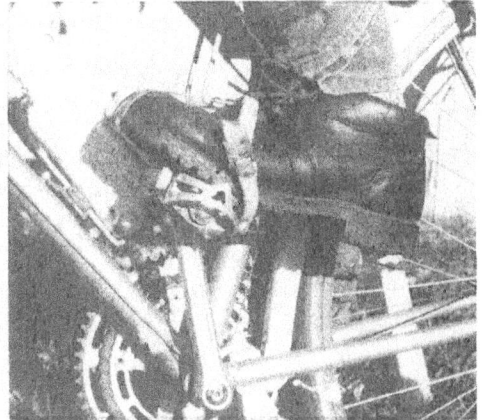

only will the thigh and calf muscles be used for propulsion, but those in the foot arch will assist by adding the mechanical fulcrum action. This technique and the straps combine to help 'pull' the pedal upward in the next stroke; the result is the greatest possible application of musculature to the task.

In short, you should leave the bike shop with 'rat-trap' pedals (ridged edges on the pedal surface to assist in slip prevention), pedals which break down to allow ball-bearing maintenance, and pedals with toeclips and straps attached. (In Part Two I'll describe the technique of getting into your toeclips easily during city riding.)

Wheels

Our last subject before we leave the bike shop is wheels, the circular metal hoops which are connected to the hubs by spokes, and covered on the outside by tires. When someone says 'wheel' in the shop, the entire apparatus of rim (the metal hoop which holds the tire), hub, axle, spokes, and tire is brought to mind. For the rider who expects to commute and take cross-country rides, the wheel as it is found on a medium price range bike in the shop should be just fine. (Large riders with very heavy touring loads may require a thicker gauge double-butted spoke, and heavy-duty rim to add strength to the wheel.) There are many good rims on the market, and most bikes today come standard with a strong alloy rim (less expensive bikes will sport the strong but very heavy all-steel rims), which will accept either a 27 X 1.25 inch or 27 x 1 inch clincher tire.

The clincher is one of the two types of tires available, and is similar to the old automobile tires with tubes inside. When you fix a flat you'll find that over the rim rests the tape, a very thin piece of rubber or cotton which is stretched in place to protect the tube from the spokes which come up through the rim base. Then comes the inner tube, of either regular or heavy weight. For now, make sure you specify in the shop that you wish "puncture-resistant" or "thorn-proof tubes in place of the regular ones. (I'll discuss the reasons in a moment.) Following the tube is the tire - called a 'clincher' if it is made for use with a tube and possesses a metal beading along the inside. When stretched around the rim this bead clinches or holds fast upon the wheel. (Later I'll teach you a trick a gentleman outside London taught me in '74 - how to fold a clincher in such a manner as to keep from injuring the metal beading, and making it small enough to carry an extra tire on long tours.) Most clinchers come with Schrader-type tube valves - just like valves on cars. The second type of tire comes with a Presta valve, which prohibits you from borrowing a little air from the corner gas station unless you have an inexpensive screw-on converter.

This second type of tire is called a tubular (or 'sew-up' - from the necessary method of repair after a flat). The tire and tube are one, like most car tires today. It has no metal beading, weighs very little, and can hold a bit more air pressure than the clincher. (The greater the air pressure the easier it is to pedal.) But the tubular pays a price for its advantages. Punctures are more common, and repairs are a very lengthy process. Especially now, when manufacturers are coming out with increasingly narrow clinchers to reduce road friction, and with the ability to hold almost as much pressure as tubulars, I cannot see why anyone would opt for the hassle of tubulars for commuting and touring.

To be fair, however, I should admit to arguments with other riders over this issue - two riders in particular who never tour with packs and tents and sleeping bags, but are interested only in covering ground quickly. And I suppose they have a valid point, if you aren't commuting and touring with the usual loads of twenty to thirty pounds. But let me tell you why, even for long-distance rides, I choose heavy clinchers and puncture-resistant tubes.

On our round-the-world ride in '74, Wayne Hartmann and I had twenty-five flats. Twenty-four of them came while we were using regular-weight (much thinner than the puncture-resistant) tubes, and only one after we had gone to the PR (or TR) tubes. With the idea of reducing our rolling weight we had opted for the regular tubes, and had the usual number of punctures (the British term for flats) - a couple apiece in Ohio and Virginia, a few in the British Isles and Western Europe, a few more behind the Iron Curtain and on through Greece, Palestine, and Africa. And a high point of four in one day in India. On through Asia, and we became hopeful that when we got to the States the better roads would mean fewer flats. Back home, we headed out through the Santa Monica Mountains for the final leg of our trip. But we didn't get far. With the first flat, we pulled the tubes, pumped them up to listen for the air escaping from the hole, and to our dismay heard the noise in a half-dozen places. Tiny cactus needles, invisible to us as we rode along, had worked their way through the tires to attack us. They cost us a day, but we learned a good lesson. Limping back into Los Angeles, we purchased four PR tubes, and slapped them in place. The following morning we pedalled through the mountains and cactus needles without difficulty, and had only one flat during the remaining 2,000 miles of our ride. We were sold. Since then I have always travelled with PR tubes and clincher tires. The time and hassle saved with fewer flats more than makes up for the small loss of pedalling ease.

I mentioned the different size of tires. Most ten-speeds today are standard as far as wheel diameter - 27 inches - but vary in the tire width with 1 1/4 , 1 1/8, and 1 inch sizes available. Rolling speed is greatest with the most narrow tire, but again I choose the largest (and therefore heaviest) for commuting. My choice is made for reasons of traction - since I ride my cycle in all kinds of weather I want as much rubber on the road as possible, even if it is going to slow me down a bit. Especially for commuting my suggestion is clincher tires, 27 x 1 V4 , with PR tubes. And don't buy any tires with a suggested inflation pressure of less than 80 pounds. (I bet this figure surprised those of you who are used to car tires only - for they carry but 28 to 32 pounds pressure on average.) I normally ride with tires of 90 pounds air pressure per square inch (p.s.i), and check them at least once a week. Ride on good rubber, keep them pumped up to where they belong, and you won't have to worry about punctures. I've had two in the last nine thousand miles of commuting and touring, and both only cost me a ten minute repair job.

Finally, unless you are purchasing a very expensive mount I would stay away from hubs with sealed bearings. Such set-ups require a special tool for cone adjustment (which you'll learn about in Part Two), and are therefore good on long tours only if they can be trusted to last.

Well, it took us a while, but we're out of the bike shop. You haven't finished gathering together all the things you need for your bike, such as luggage racks and fenders and a lighting system, but these are things which you can add yourself, and save a few dollars by doing so. As for the basic machine you are now set up with a mount which will take you to the corner pub or around the world and back. Clothing is yet to come, and riding techniques, touring and commuting tips, and some suggestions for planning long rides. Before I launch into those subjects, however, I'll give you a checklist of all the items we've just gone through, so you'll have an easy time refreshing your memory before heading for the shop.

Checklist

Frame

1. *Size* - be sure the bike 'fits' you, both in height and length. Straddle the bike, but don't sit on the saddle. Stand Hat-footed in the lowest-heeled shoes you think you'll ride in, and pull up on the handlebars - slowly. You should have a clearance of about V2 inch. Less, and you stand the chance of coming off the saddle and racking yourself on the top tube. More, and you'll have to find an extra-long seat post to allow for leg extension. (Frame height is

measured from the middle of the bottom bracket to the top of the seat tube; standard frames are 19", 21", 23", 25", and 27".) That takes care of the height. Now stand alongside the bike, and place your arm in front of the saddle parallel to the top tube. Your elbow should just touch the nose or front tip of the saddle, your hand will extend toward the handlebars. If the bike fits you as far as length is concerned your finger-tips will reach a point roughly between the handlebar stem and the handlebar itself. This will insure that when riding your hands will easily reach the brakes. Many people complain of sore backs, tired arms and neck muscles long after such discomfort should have passed. The reason is that the bike is too long for them. But don't toss your old bike away just yet, if this is the case with you. There are solutions short of a new machine, and less painful than lengthening your arms. First, the bottom of the saddle is made to compensate for differences in arm length, by loosening the holding bolt and sliding the saddle forward a bit. Second, you can tilt your handlebars up slightly, as I prefer, so that your brakes are a bit higher on the 'curl' of the bar, thereby lessening the distance from the saddle. Third, handlebars are made with different bar extensions - that is, the length of the juncture between stem and bar. Even if the salesman fails to measure you in this way, be sure to do so yourself. Your comfort and riding efficiency depend upon it. And once you think you've found the bike that fits you, take it out for a test ride.

2. *Lugs* - remember that lugs don't always mean a stronger frame, but they usually do. They can cover up a lousy job of tube connection of the cheap models. If the lugs look a bit sloppy on the outside ask the salesman to remove the seat post. Then, reach into the frame with your finger and feel for the mitering. It should be smooth and straight. A very expensive bike with precise mitering and larger than usual tubes may be strong without lugs. But in a medium price range of $250 - $400 you should look for lugs. Every bike I've had in the last fifteen years has been lugged.

3. *Double-butted* - extra strength, less weight. But not a necessity as far as I'm concerned. The bike I took around the world had only straight-gauge tubing, but its good lugs and internal construction made it strong.

4. *Fork-rake/wheel base* - buy a touring fork for comfort if you don't plan to race. and get a bike with a long wheel base for the same reason. If the salesman doesn't know if the wheel base is long or short then you're in the wrong shop.

5. *Frame composition* - like the double-butted choice, your wallet decides this issue. I have one of the best now, 531 Reynolds, but again it was the motorist who hit me and her insurance company who got me into that league. Before then it was a strong but heavier frame. If it was my money I'd spend less and lose a few ounces off the engine - me. But, don't buy a bike weighing 30 pounds or more -stay in the mid-to-upper twenty pound range.
6. *Frame style* - strongest of all is the men's. Mixtes are fine for rough commuting and touring with light loads. Women's models are out.

Crank

1. *Cotteriess* - end of discussion. Buy a cotterpin system and you deserve the maintenance hassle you get.

2. *Five-pin crankarm* - not a three-pin. Buy a five-pin and you'll have less play side-to-side in your chain-ring.

3. *Interchangeable crankarm/chainrings* - get a system which allows you to switch chainrings without having to buy a new right side crankarm. Most systems are built this way.

Gearing

1. *Chain rings* -1 ride with a 54 tooth large, 42 small. My wife handles a 52-40. Don't let the salesman tell you a 52-47 is a wide enough range for anything but the Alps. It isn't. *You* are going to climb the hills, not him. So *you* decide.

2. *Freewheel* - my wife and I both ride with 14-34 free-wheels. As above, this is a very wide touring range which I don't have to be climbing mountains to appreciate. Another idea is a 52-38 front, and a 14-30 rear. I suggest this as an alternative because several bikes come equipped now with derailleurs which have a capacity of only 30 teeth for the cluster. By dropping the small chainring up front to a 38 you still gain a wider range, and in fact reduce the bike's weight a few ounces. Still, I prefer the 14-34 freewheel, as it allows me to commute entirely on the larger chainring up front.

Derailleurs

1. *Which kind?* - I'm not worried about you getting stuck with a lousy set of changers (another name for derailleur) as long as you de-mand the wide range in gearing, for any derailleur that can handle

that range is well made. Sun Tour puts out an inexpensive front and rear changer set which is pleasing to the eye and works like a champ. I had eight years on my VGT without a bit of trouble.

Shifters

1. *Location* - my preference is on the down tube. I also do not care for the ratchet shifters, for they are noisy and more apt to break on tour.

Quick-release

1. *Necessary?* - not a requirement for me, but surely an appreciated convenience.

Handlebars

1. *Drop-bars* - for all my reasons before - give these a chance.

2. *Position* - your bars should sit no lower than one inch below the top of your saddle. Be sure the handlebar stem is long enough for this adjustment.

Saddle

1. *Which kind?* - don't buy a mattress type. After that, my preference is leather. Avocet and Bikecology have "anatomic" saddles which promise greater comfort. Your choice.

Brakes

1. *Which kind?* - again your choice except in the very inexpensive line, where I opt for the center-pull to give more even braking.

2. *Hooded brake levers* - a real must. If you don't believe me go ride fifty miles with your hands over metal brakes and we'll talk again. Also good for insulating your hands from the cold metal in winter.

Pedals

1. *Maintenance* - you can go for years without having problems with pedals which are not made to allow simple bearing maintenance, but I like the idea of riding my last mile fifty years from now with the same pedals I use today. Your choice, but for me it's a few extra dollars for a set I can take apart with ease.

2. *Reflectors* - one of the best safety features on a bike is the tiny reflector at the back of each pedal. Be sure you have them.

3. *Fit* - check out the pedals for all size as far as width is concerned. This is especially important for those pedals which turn up at the edge, and for those riders who plan to tour or commute in winter with boots.

4. Toeclips and straps - definitely. And give yourself time to get used to them.

Wheels

1. *Clinchers* - stay clear of tubulars unless you plan to race, and possess the patience of my grandmother.

2. *Tubes* - puncture resistant, Schrader valve.

3. *Tires* - at least 80 pounds per square inch air pressure, and preferably higher. Stay with either 1V4 or 1 1/8 in width so that you'll handle the PR tubes.

4. *Spokes* - unless you are an exceptionally large rider, the spokes in standard wheels should do nicely. If you are worried, you might ask a good shop to replace the standard wheels with a heavy gauge double-butted spoke and a heavy rim. While discussing wheels you will hear the terms 'three-cross' and 'four-cross' - references to the number of spokes any single spoke crosses from the hub to the rim. (Generally a four-cross will denote a longer spoke, and therefore a somewhat softer ride.) Spoke length is partially determined by the lace pattern, but is more directly a result of having either 'high-flange' hubs (wider, and thus shorter spokes), or 'low flange' hubs (less wide, and therefore longer spokes).

5. *Hubs* - no 'sealed bearings' unless you are buying very expensive wheels.

We haven't discussed the following items yet, but I'll add them to the checklist here for easy reference.

Fenders

1. Take a ride without them on wet streets and you'll spend the day at work with a streak up your back. Front fender keeps your feet from getting wet, and both protect brakes from road grit. Bluemels and Esge are two good names in very light-weight, yet durable, plastic fenders.

Safety Hag

1. Increases a rider's visibility tremendously. Great on the open road and in city traffic. A must. There are now side-mount safety flags available, which are designed to keep cars from coming too close as they pass. The theory is fine, but my experience tells me the pretty orange side flag would be too great a temptation for the occasional idiot on the rider's side of the car. Most would avoid it, a few would slap at it, but only one would have to grab for it to cause an accident. Stay with the flag which mounts at the axle and flies a foot over your head.

Reflectors

1. Most bike shops load you up with them - one in front and one rear, and one in the spokes of either wheel. Again, make sure they are on both pedals.

Luggage racks

1. Makes your cycle a true tool for transporting something besides just your body. I have one front and rear. (See later chapters for further discussion.) Also, choose a frame which has single or double 'eyelets' near the dropouts, to make rack and fender attachment easier and more secure.

Water bottle

1. One water bottle in its 'cage' (bottle mount) is necessary even for city riding. Not that you'll be all that thirsty around town, but I carry straight ammonia in mine for dogs that ail me, and motorists with big mouths and loud horns.

Lighting

1. Every model has its drawbacks. Batteries run down and throw a poor beam, generators cause wheel drag and go off when you aren't pedalling. But I opt for the Schwinn LeTour rear-mounted generator set. It has both tail and headlight, provides a good beam, and produces only minimum wheel drag.

When friends are in the market for a bike I usually suggest they look at the following choices. Don't limit your choices to these, of course, but do compare them with the competition.

Fuji (Royale) 12 speed

frame - lugged, chrome molybdenum, straight gauge (main tubes) brakes - Dia Compe 500 G side-pull gearing - cotterless crank (52-42 front, 14-30 rear) derailleurs - Sun Tour (front - Road VX, rear - Road VX-S) weight - 27 pounds cost - $325

Trek (412) 12 speed

frame - lugged, Ishiwata 022 chrome molybdenum, doublebutted (main tubes)

brakes - Dia Compe 500 side-pull gearing - cotterless crank (52-40 front, 14-30 rear) derailleurs - Sun Tour (front - Road VX, rear - Road VX-GT) weight - 25 pounds cost - $339

Schwinn (Voyageur) 12 speed

frame - lugged, chrome molybdenum main tubes, top and down tubes double-butted

brakes - Dia Compe 500 G side-pull gearing - cotterless crank (52-40 front, 13-28 rear) derailleurs - Shimano Altus LT weight - 25 V2 pounds cost - $350

Fuji (S-12-S SL) 12 speed

frame - lugged, double-butted chrome molybdenum (main tubes) brakes - Dia Compe 500 G side-pull gearing - cotterless crank (52-42 front, 14-30 rear) derailleurs - Sun Tour (front - Road VX, rear - Road VXS) weight - 25 pounds cost - $380

Part Two
Commuting

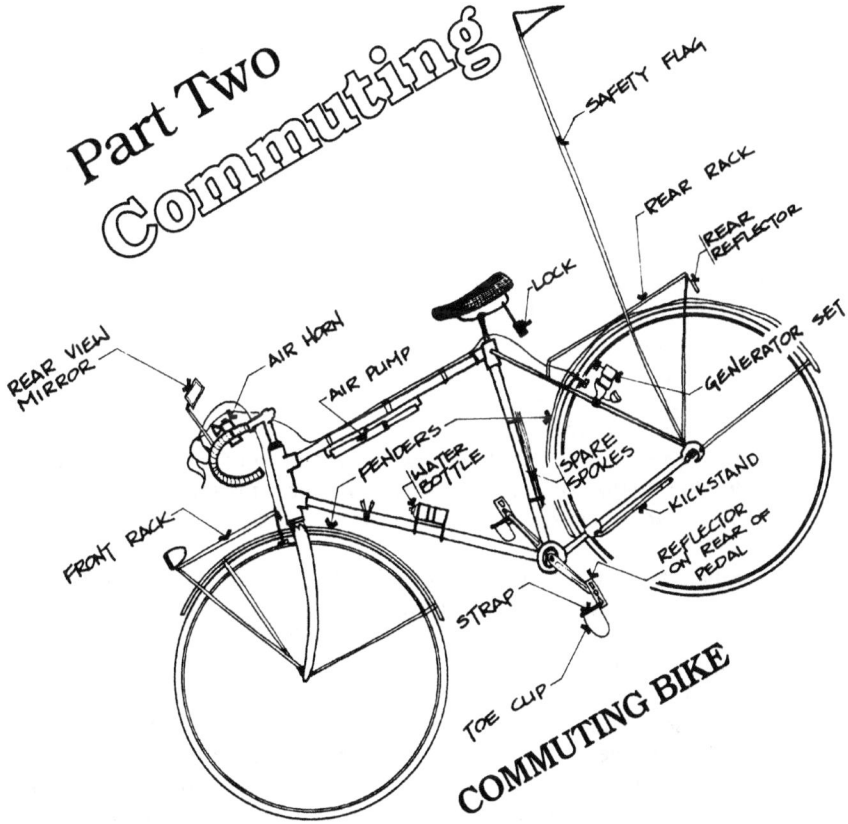

SAFETY FLAG

REAR RACK

REAR REFLECTOR

LOCK

GENERATOR SET

REAR VIEW MIRROR

AIR HORN

AIR PUMP

FENDERS

WATER BOTTLE

SPARE SPOKES

KICKSTAND

FRONT RACK

REFLECTOR ON REAR OF PEDAL

STRAP

TOE CLIP

COMMUTING BIKE

T HE snowstorm had hit the city at three a.m., and by rush hour that morning six inches of white fluff covered the streets. I had left home early, allowing myself twice the normal time it took to get to work. Stocking cap, goggles, warm gloves and water-proofed light-weight hiking boots all combined to keep me comfortable in the cold. I pedalled along the streets with little trouble, for my narrow bike tires cut through the snow to make good traction with the road below.

In the block ahead of me I could see a huge Buick spinning its wheels at a forty-five degree angle to the curb. Its wide tires had compressed the snow beneath them, and now sat slipping on top. I pedalled alongside and knocked on the car door. The lady behind the wheel rubbed off enough of the window fog with her gloved hand to let me see her eyes first take in my snow-covered hat and goggles, then unbelievingly drop to see me straddling my bicycle. I yelled over the engine noise.

"Need some help?"

Slowly the window cranked down, but the woman didn't answer my question. Instead came words which fit her expression of disbelief.

"You must be crazy," she said slowly, "to ride a bicycle in this weather!"

I smiled, reminding myself that I was, after all, talking to a motorist.

"Yes ma'am," I replied, "But at least I'm moving."

That true story illustrates the amazing difficulty people have in imagining getting to and from work on a bike. For many of them the notion has never come up, or if it has the unthinking response was 'oh, that's something they do in England, not here.' Most people simply have not viewed commuting by bike as a viable alternative to the automobile. That's unfortunate. But these chapters should show you how wrong they are. And, they will help you to avoid the mistakes my wife and I made when we began riding to work in 1975.

There are three primary factors in commuting by bicycle - comfort, safety, and mechanics. You've already learned how to buy a bike which fits you comfortably, but remaining dry in the rain and warm when it's cold is also a necessity. The presence of so many cars on the road makes safe, defensive riding a requirement just to stay alive. And, although your bike will never refuse to start in the morning, you should still get to know it mechanically to keep it running at its best. Commuting by bike will be easiest, least expensive, and most enjoyable when you're an expert in all these areas.

2. Commuting in Comfort

Rain

You will recall that I suggested fenders for your bike in Chapter One. They will keep a good amount of road water from splashing up on you, but you'll still have to deal with getting wet from rain. Back in '74 when Wayne and I took off on our long tour we made the mistake of planning for rainy days by buying two-piece rain suits. These were well-made outfits with reinforced seams and snaps and drawstring closures to seal us hermetically from the outer world. And they were perfect for the cold rains we encountered in early summer riding in Ireland, and again when crossing the Rockies the following winter. But all the while between, when the temperatures were above 50 degrees F., riding in the suits produced as much moisture inside through perspiration as that present outside in the form of rain. Therefore, let me suggest a cooler alternative - the poncho.

I can already hear the moans from those of you who are veterans, and have memories of soggy days spent patrolling in the mud. wearing a thick and heavy green Army poncho that was too long to let you walk easily, and just short enough to allow the rain inside the tops of your boots. But stop the crying, for again progress has been made in creating the happy biker. Today's bicycle ponchos are light-weight, compress into envelope size, and are cut to allow easy pedalling. And not only will the poncho keep your upper half dry, but your legs and feet as well, if the rain is not coming down at an extreme angle.

Take a close look at the poncho and you'll notice how this rainwear is adapted for the bike. First, the backside is made to tie about your waist, allowing protection for your rear. The front half has thumb loops on the inside, which allow the rider to stretch the front all the way to the handlebars, still keeping the fingers free for braking and shifting gears. This arrangement makes possible a tent-like protection for legs and feet beneath, and for air to flow under the poncho to cool the rider and cut down on perspiration. The neck has two snaps to facilitate removal, and as another means to allow air to circulate under the poncho. Finally, a hood is available to keep the head dry.

I have had one problem with the poncho during rainstorms. Gusts of wind will occasionally cause the sleeve folds to flap about, and therefore allow rain to get inside. This can be alleviated by sewing a snap or piece of velcro on either side of the poncho flap which serves as a sleeve. When this is done I find the poncho almost as impervious to rain as the more expensive rain jackets, and far preferable due to the circulation of air permitted.

As I mentioned above, when rain comes in from the side it can get past the tent-like protection which the poncho allows. In this case it is necessary to protect the lower torso and feet. Again, this can be done with a two-piece rainsuit such as that which I used for so long. But, as with the jacket, rain pants are extremely hot to wear. Today I tour cross-country in all seasons and commute throughout the year with a poncho on top and rain chaps, rather than pants, beneath. Chaps cover merely the leg, not the trunk. Therefore, they are to be used with a poncho only, not a rain jacket, for the jacket will not keep your lower trunk dry. Chaps tie onto the belt loops of your trousers, or can attach by lengthening the tie strings and looping them around your thigh.

Now you are dry from head to ankle, and we have only the feet left to cover. In the last year several sportswear outfitters have marketed what are unfortunately called 'rain booties'. These are somewhat similar to the old-style galoshes we wore as kids, except that they are made of gore-tex or some other light-weight material. The 'booties' cover the entire foot, and extend up the leg about nine inches - a combination boot-gaiter. (More terms! Gaiters are coverings for the instep, ankle, and sometimes calf of the leg. If you're an old drum-major you know them as spats; if you're a vet you call them leggings, and if you are over a hundred you probably know them as 'puttees'.) Gore tex is a man-made fabric which allows a piece of apparel to be rainproof and yet 'breathable' at the same time. That is, a rainsuit of gore-tex will keep you dry both ways - no rain coming in, and the air which is warmed by your body passing out of the fabric. This is possible due to the great difference in size between a rain droplet and a water vapor molecule. The material has thousands of tiny holes far too small to let rain pass, but large enough to let the water vapor -perspiration - escape. Only two problems with a gore-tex rainsuit: first, you have to keep them fairly clean, or the tiny holes plug up and you're back to wearing a plastic bag. And secondly, a rainsuit of this stuff costs over a hundred dollars - five times the cost of the poncho and chaps. Yak Works offers an entire gore-tex rainsuit; jacket - $120, chaps - $69, hood - $17. Rain booties are nice, and I'd like to buy a pair. But I'll have to wait until I get hit again for some motorist to buy them for me, for they cost between $40 and $70. My entire lower-half set up (chaps and overshoes) cost me less than half that. (Bike Warehouse; poncho and chaps - $22.50, rubber shoe covers $6.45.)

Several years ago I bought a pair of light-weight rubber overshoes called 'Totes'. They are just like the more expensive 'booties' except that they have no easy-access zipper arrangement, and the top is flared, with no draw-string closure as on the high-priced models. But they've worked just fine for me as long as I pull the chaps' cuffs over them, to keep the rain out. (Don't get the low-topped overshoes, the ones which merely cover the shoes and not the ankle as well. Be sure to buy the ones which extend up the leg a bit.)

Okay, you're dressed for the monsoons. But before we leave this topic let me tell you how I've changed my rain riding habits in the last year - just as a second option for you. The poncho remains, and the chaps are along for the ride in case the wind picks up a bit (stored nicely in my bike bag for easy access). But instead of the overshoes and chaps for protection I've found that a pair of high gaiters worn with my well-oiled light-weight hiking boots have been sufficient to ward off the droplets in all but the worst of storms. (Naturally, such boots would be too hot for summer, so chaps and Totes remain for warm weather.) The gaiters fit around the instep, cover the ankle and calf, and protect the entire tongue-closure of the boot top. The only portion of the boot left open to rain is the lower shell above the sole -the critical junction for water penetration. This area is impermeable when treated generously with Sno-Seal, saddle soap, or the leather dressing of your choice. (REI: $1.50 $3.00) Thus my feet are kept dry by my boots, my ankles and calves covered by the gaiters, my thighs, torso, arms and head protected by the poncho. When I get to work it's a quick change of merely removing the poncho like a T-shirt, and unzipping the gaiters. (If you decide to try this be sure to buy gaiter switch zip or snap in front of the leg, not behind. It's much easier.)

A final note on rain pants or chaps. Whichever you choose, be sure to get the legs long enough still to cover your ankle when pedalling. Don't buy them if they fit you like a pair of suitpants, for they'll ride up and expose your lower leg to the rain. This is the problem Wayne and I had in '74. Our rain pants too short, and our shoe tops not high enough to span the gap, we tried to fashion gaiters to protect the leg between. Plastic bread bags appeared to be the least expensive choice so we cut out the closed end and slipped them onto our legs, then bloused the bottoms over the shoe tops. We looked like clowns with our bright bread bag-gaiters as we pedalled through England. But we were dry.

Some other rain-riding tips

Your poncho or jacket hood will keep your head dry, but won't do much to keep the rain out of your eyes. During a normal shower I find little difficulty in seeing properly, but a single droplet hitting the eyeball itself really hurts. To escape this I slip on the pair of sunglasses I always have with me in my bike bag. Too dark? Then invest in a pair of photo-gray lenses which lighten up when little sun is present. Or slip on the goggles which you carry in your bag, or rather will carry, if you follow my directions for snow-riding. (Sunglasses - REI, EMS; $8.50 -$30. Goggles - REI, EMS; $4.50 - $9)

Carry a bandana with you. Highly absorbent, it will dry in no time when stretched over a radiator or heating vent, or in the sun if the weather changes. Takes up almost no space in a pannier.

You'll notice an increased awareness of the weather once you

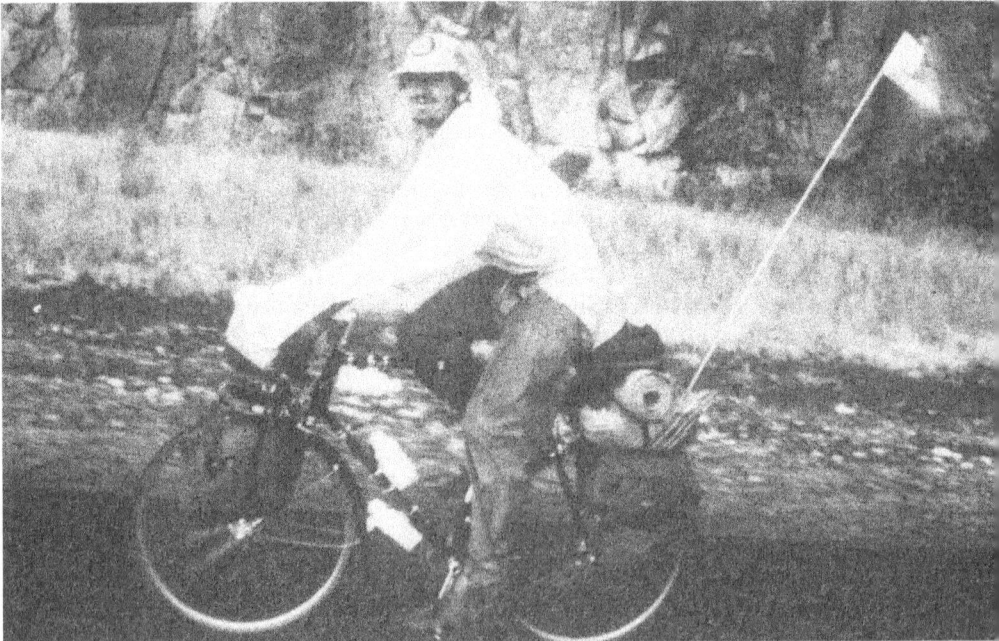

begin riding regularly, and after a while an ability to predict rain in plenty of time to dismount and suit up. You'll notice a change in wind direction, a fresh smell to the air, perhaps the sighting of showers in the distance, or rain on cars coming toward you, often with their headlights on. Be observant, and you'll stay dry.

Travel side roads even more than usual to avoid the drenching splashes by passing cars.

Realize that with a little planning, a biker can be dryer after a ten mile ride to work than a motorist who sprints from the parking lot to his office.

And, finally, knowing that you are impervious to the rain, learn to enjoy and even look forward to the different sights, subdued sounds and fresh smells of rainy days.

Snow and Cold Weather Gear

I must admit at the beginning that I take a special pleasure in winter touring and commuting. There are many reasons for this, but the two most important are these: first, I like having the road to myself on occasion, for all the fair-weather riders are off the road from October to April; and secondly, I am honestly more comfortable riding in the winter. This is something motorists have a terrible time understanding, and generally refuse to believe even after I give all the reasons. Just as you will remain dry in your poncho-chaps-overshoes outfit, you will be warm if you follow the tips my wife and I can give you after many unfortunately cold rides. Comfort also comes from the fact that in winter a rider can adjust his body warmth by adding or discarding a layer of clothing, and by changing pedalling speed. In summer one can finally get down to bare skin to cool off, but no further. So on to the first tip: layering, which has subtly changed the way we dress both on the road and around town.

When I had a car and when it was cold outside I threw on a heavy parka or Army field jacket before leaving the house. This coat kept me from freezing until the car heater warmed up, and then it could be adjusted for comfort. Now that the car is gone the parka and heavy coats have had to remain in the closet, for they are almost useless on a bike. Their warmth may be appreciated for the first three blocks or so, but after this - when the body's heater has begun to work through exercise - they are too warm. Even when unzipped they provide too much insulation. If removed entirely the result is too extreme, especially if any perspiration has appeared. The wind would then hit and produce a chill, which might convince you to put the coat back on, and the process would be repeated. Another problem: such coats are far too cumbersome to put inside a pannier, and thus would remain exposed to rain or snow while attached to your rear carrier. Finally, a poncho worn over a parka during a winter rain produces even more heat, and more perspiration.

The solution for me is a light-weight jacket on top, and only my regular shirt and tie and undershirt beneath. On very cold days, or when the wind-chill is great, I add a long-sleeve sweater or pullover insulated underwear top beneath the jacket. On such days, if I become too warm it is only a minute's stop to pull off the jacket and slip in into a pannier. Five miles later if I am too warm, again off comes the sweater, or the jacket is replaced if too cold, or the jacket in place of the sweater if a different temperature is desired. By such 'layering' a rider can adjust his clothing to facilitate almost any weather change and will be prepared to act quickly to forestall perspiration.

This sounds like a real bother, the changing of layers all the time. And if it were done all the time it would be a pain. But after a few cold rides to work, you'll get to know just about the right number and kinds of layers to start off with. (The most I have to do in winter for warmth is add the insulated underwear, or to cool off just unzip the jacket front. Spring brings on a switch of the jacket for a windbreaker; summer brings on a switch to a loin cloth, et. cetera.) I might add that the new government suggested office thermostat settings will bring about layering as well. Once again there will be a reason for vested suits other than mere style.

I have mentioned the jacket only to illustrate the point of layering, and will now describe my winter wardrobe in detail, moving from headgear on down to boots and socks.

Head

Several times in past years while reading articles on backpacking I've seen sentences similar to this: 'The body is like a furnace, with the head serving a chimney. Fail to cover your head with a hat in winter and you lose 70% of body heat.' I've always found this notion interesting, but never have I seen an explanation of why this is true, or how the 70% figure is derived. But proof or not, my own experience is that in cold weather I cannot be warm without good headgear. In fact, I ride with a hat for three of the four seasons, and even carry a hat with me on summer tours for early morning and late evening rides at high altitudes.

My preference for winter commuting is a heavy stocking cap pulled over a full head of hair. (On fall or spring mornings I opt for the 'sports cap', the English model with the snap in front. L.L. Bean, $10 - $16.) By full head I'm not referring to length, but to thickness of hair. You'll think this is silly, but beginning in September I utilize the insulating qualities of thick hair by not allowing the barber's 'thinner' scissors to approach my scalp. The length of hair doesn't seem to matter, except on summer tours when I find any hair too hot, beyond that small amount necessary to shield me from the sun. As with vests, bike commuters will quickly begin to see beyond 'style'.

I like a wool stocking cap (REI, EMS; $1.50 - $4.95) for its warmth even when wet, and its versatility as far as amount of head covered. When not too cold it remains rolled up on top the head; when frigid it easily covers the ears. There are various thicknesses of stocking caps, but I would opt for a very thick wool cap if I were buying just one. (Note: I have found no practical value whatever to the ball on top of so many caps. I must admit, though, to its certain aesthetic quality. Whether this offsets the additional weight factor of perhaps 60 grams or so is up to the individual rider.)

You bikers who live in areas where snow-skiing is not big may have a difficult time finding goggles except in catalogues. If your climate produces only occasional light snow showers you can get by with the sunglasses you already have for hard rains. But goggles are a necessity for big-flake areas, and should, with your stocking cap, have a permanent winter position in your ever-present commuting bike bag. (An inexpensive alternative to ski goggles, and one which I prefer due to cost and smaller size, is the EMS Glacier goggle - $4.75.)

Just this winter my wife gave up her scarf for what is called a 'neck-gaiter' (REI $4.25). This is a small cuff of material which resembles a detached turtle-neck, and serves the same function. It is slipped over the head into place around the neck, and there may remain rolled once to cover only an exposed area of skin, or may be unfurled so as to protect the neck and lower chin from cold winds. In commuting I require neither of these (gaiter or turtle-neck shirts), though my wife uses the gaiter in very cold weather.

This takes care of the head from the top and ears to the neck, but what of the face between? Granted, not much skin remains; the forehead and ears are covered by the cap, eyes by goggles, neck and chin by gaiter or scarf. Only the nose and cheeks are exposed. I have dealt with part of this by growing a full beard. The high cheek and nose are still exposed, but this has never bothered me while commuting, and only once while touring - crossing the Rockies in November. On that occasion I merely donned a pullover ski-mask. If you live in Minnesota or some other clime with frigid winter temperatures, you may opt for a ski-mask or balaclava (headgear similar to the ski-mask but usually with a stiffened visor) when the wind-chill is great, or rub a small amount of vaseline on your nose or cheeks. (I have never been forced by temperature extremes in five winters to do this, though I have tried it to see the effect. My vaselined skin felt warmer while riding, and rubbed off easily with my bandana when I got to work.) 'Wind-chill' refers to the effects of wind in cold weather;

air temperature and wind velocity combine to produce a much lower equivalent temperature. For example, on a day when the temperature is 10 degrees F. and the wind is approximately 20 miles per hour the equivalent wind-chill temperature is minus 32 degrees F. And if you are riding in wet conditions the equivalent wind-chill is -74 degrees F! Weather forecasts in areas with extreme ranges of cold temperatures will often warn of the dangers of human flesh freezing. Again, I have never had to worry while commuting. But on winter tours I carry both a ski-mask and a small tube of vaseline.

Upper Torso

Unless you have ridden in cold weather you are probably still having difficulty with the idea that a jogger or biker in the dead of winter can actually be warm wearing so little clothing. But on almost every winter day I leave the house with only undershirt, dress shirt, tie, and light jacket as covering for my upper body. My wife wears the same with the exception of a camisole in place of an undershirt, though normally this too is not worn except on quite cold days. Wool or flannel shirts provide the necessary added warmth on days when the temperature is in the low-teens, but even then I shun the heavy pull-over sweaters which are so nice for walking in such weather. In fact, I stay away from almost all pullover clothing (aside from insulated underwear), for I can't open the neck or front as I might wish to prevent perspiration once the riding has made me warm. The warm bulky sweaters are passed over for the same reason as the heavy coats - the preference for light-weight layerings of clothing.

The material and cut of the jacket is thus extremely important, for this outer garment must be versatile enough to carry you warmly from October until April, and yet not cause too great a heat build-up when under a poncho during rains or wet snows. The best jacket I've found thus far has a shell made of 50% cotton and 50% polyester, and a single thin-layer sewn-in lining of 65% polyester, 35% cotton. It is breathable, and yet warm due to its wind-stopping features of snap-closure cuffs, drawstring waist, high-zip neck, and full length -extending ten to twelve inches below my waist. This last feature prevents exposure of the small of my back when in the crouch-riding position, as takes place with short jackets. Along this line of proper fitting, the sleeves should be longer than normal so as to still cover wrists when arms are outstretched to the handlebars. And the jacket should fit loosely enough to allow another layer beneath, or a great amount of cooling air to circulate when desired. (My wife's winter jacket has an additional advantage here - a double zipper which allows her to unzip from the bottom up. This gives even greater control over air-flow, and provides for easy leg movement.) Finally, four large pockets provide ample space for gloves or cap if I should want to remove them while riding and not stop to put them in a pannier. My jacket is white, for visibility at night. And it is made to be machine-washed and dried. (I haven't found this coat in any of the usual sports catalogues, as their coats are generally heavier and made of more 'exotic' fabrics. My jacket cost $24 - check J.C. Penneys, Sears, and similar stores.)

Hands

Along with feet, hands are the most difficult portion of the body to keep warm. But the problem can be solved by purchasing an expensive pair of gloves, and by using a front handlebar bag as a windbreak with a lighter and less expensive pair. (Remember the discussion of wind-chill.)

Until last year, when my wife gave me a birthday present of the warmest gloves I've ever had, I wore a wool liner-leather shell set-up. You vets will remember this from the service, and my combination was similar except that the leather shells had cuffs which extended over my wrist and up the arm for several inches. Three times a year I treated the leather with one of the dressings I've mentioned earlier, and used my awl to restitch any separating seams (sewing awls - REI, EMS; $3.75, instructions included)- On warm days I would remove the wool liner, taking advantage of the layers of gloves. But there was the problem, encountered perhaps no more than twenty times over the past five years, of the wool and leather simply not adding up to enough insulation to prevent my hands from becoming painfully cold. On such frigid days I would strap on my handlebar bag, and hold the bars in such a place that the wind did not strike my hands directly. This was sufficient, until my wife gave me a pair of the expensive downhill ski gloves. The man-made filler insulates beautifully; the warm sock-like wrist covering is tight-fitting and extends half-way up my forearm. (Name brand is Grandoe - REI; $34.)

Therefore, I suggest the best pair of gloves your wallet can buy. I also suggest that you forego mittens, even though they can be warmer due to the heat produced by all fingers being together. Mittens reduce a rider's manual dexterity to the point of danger when grabbing for a brake lever in an emergency. Finally, be sure that your gloves have a durable water-repellent leather shell, keep them that way with periodic dressings, and learn to use a leather awl to deal with the small rips before they become large tears.

Lower Torso

I am still, fifteen years later, embarrassed by the memory. It was my first long tour, and Roy and I had planned for it meticulously; $60 each to cover expenses of three weeks on the road (it was 1965), two pairs of riding shorts (no long pants at all), windbreakers sprayed with a waterproofing chemical rather than ponchos or rainsuits (this was my father's idea). The money just made it, but only by four days on a diet of beans and bread. The waterproofed windbreakers held out the rain for the first five minutes, and then transformed themselves into sponges. And the lack of long pants, which we had thought unnecessary because it was June? Well, as early as Iowa the temperature made us part with one-sixth of our cash reserves to buy insulated underwear. Without enough money to buy long pants in addition we were forced to pedal through the northern states and around Canada with the lower half of our long-Johns showing. And, near the end of the 1,700 mile trek, the bottoms of our shorts began to wear thin, for we hadn't chosen the material with any knowledge of such things. Had the journey been five hundred miles further we would have been riding in long-Johns alone.

I relate that touring story in this commuting section because it gives two lessons for any cold weather riding: choose a durable trouser material so the bottoms won't disappear, and wear long-Johns beneath them. We Americans have spent three decades driving in warm cars to heated offices and factories. The only long underwear we've seen, aside from hunters' and skiiers', have been the one-piece red outfits on cowboys in the movies. But this is changing quickly. Bikers and non-bikers alike will find their pocketbooks dictating the change, demanding a reassessment of the function of clothing. Comfort will re-emerge over style as the first necessity. How much comfort is there in a pair of thin suitpants while standing on ice-cold car-seat vinyl in winter, or in an office when the thermostat is set at 68 degrees F? How many of you have waited for a bus in February in a suit? Biking aside, long underwear is in the cards for all of us. And now for a few pointers. Not all long-Johns are created equal. Some are warmer than others, some are bulky, some very thin. You'll have to decide for yourself on this after looking at the selection, but I can tell you that I buy the expensive "Duofold" one-or two-piece set for winter tours, and am sure to get the bottoms with legs long enough to stay in my socks. (REI; $25. This expense is justified by the quality, but for commuting alone a less expensive pair will do.) Check the label for shrinking percentages, make the salesman guarantee he'll take them back if this figure is exceeded, and then buy two pairs. You'll not wear the tops for commuting very often, but you'll need them for touring, so don't buy white long-Johns. I always buy them in colors because in a pinch, a blue or green top on a trip can double as a shirt around town; a white one only looks like you're wearing underwear in public. And now to the lesson about choosing a durable trouser material. Try to commute in all wool or corduroy, and you'll wear a patch out of your pants in a single season. I have switched to pants made of durable 11 or 12 ounce cotton duck, cotton-polyester duck material. They wear like iron (but bend more easily), and are good for all seasons. Does this mean goodbye to all the cords and thin wool suitpants? No, and there are two solutions here. First, my wife's technique is to carry her pants along folded nicely in a pannier, riding in a denim or other tough fabric which can take the wear. It only requires a minute to change when she gets to work, but it is a hassle she could omit by the second solution - a sheepskin saddle cover. I'm afraid I would feel funny strapping a furry sheepskin over my leather Brooks, but if I couldn't change at work or didn't have any very durable pants to ride in, I could probably put up with the comments. (Sheepskin seat covers - Bike Warehouse; $7.95.)

Another option. The well-made pants of heavy cotton duck are expensive - $20 - $25 per pair (REI, EMS, L.L. Bean, Sierra Designs). If you like the looks of full-polyester pants you are in luck, for these are generally inexpensive, and wear very well.

Feet

I mentioned earlier that in winter I ride with light-weight hiking boots. I slip on a thin cotton sock first, next a thick wool blend sock (all-wool tends to wear out too quickly), and then the water-proofed boots. The cold has never gotten through. My boots are the three-quarter length Muir Trail Pivettas, which have gone up from $54 three years ago to $90 today in the Ski Hut catalogue. I would not pay that amount for a light-weight boot, and therefore suggest the Fabiano #90 Madre from EMS, $66. (This is still a lot to pay, and I would check for sales of good boots in local shops and stores.) The light-weight Pivettas and Fabianos have internal stitching at the leather upper-sole junction - to produce a narrow profile which allows easy entry and exit from the toe-clips. The narrow profile also keeps the boot from making me stand out at work like a mountain climber anxious for the weekend. I wear my Pivettas all day at work, but if you prefer a regular street shoe, or are forced to don a low-cut safety shoe at your factory, then a couple of choices must be made.

First, you could do as my wife does on cold days, which is to wear the warm boots and change at work. Again, she doesn't mind this, but I would get tired and look for an alternative which could save me the trouble and time. If you decide to ride in low-quarters (regular street shoes) you can make them warm enough by the addition of gaiters to keep the wind from your ankles, and toe-clip covers to do away with the effects of wind on your feet. These are available commercially through "Polar Pals" (address in appendix), or may be home-fashioned from heavy plastic or leather. I still recommend the boots for warmth, but these alternatives do make it possible to avoid the cold. (Chances are someone will suggest that you place a thin plastic bag over your foot between the two pairs of socks. Thank them for the tip, but don't do it unless you have an extra pair of socks in your bike bag. As with the enclosed rainsuit your foot will perspire and cause considerable cold when you stop pedalling.)

Finally, you'll learn to enjoy the world at temperatures other than 72 degrees F. I don't like to be miserable, but, as with Ishmael in Moby Dick, I know the delicious enjoyment of warmth primarily because I also experience the contrast of cold - each winter's day for the first few crisp minutes of pedalling. Melville's character describes his feelings while snug in bed beneath the covers in an unheated room, "Then there you lie like the one warm spark in the heart of an arctic crystal." And there are those times in early morning in December when the drivers glance through their frosted windows, to see me enjoying the cold on my bike. 'One warm spark'. What a great description of a winter ride.

Panniers

Several times I've mentioned the need to carry your foul weather gear with you, so now we'll turn our attention to bike bags. It is my first job to convince you that with the correct panniers and the proper bicycle cart you will be able to transport everything from the month's groceries to six foot ladders to children - all without difficulty. My second task is to make you aware of the many different kinds of bags available, and their functions. Specially built bicycle panniers are a must for touring, but other bags at much lower costs will do fine for commuting. Every bike commuter needs some form of satchel to carry his foul weather gear, tools, and a few first-aid items for the occasional scrape. (Again, some terminology - the word often used for a bike bag is 'pannier', which comes from the Latin word panis, meaning 'bread', and panarium, meaning 'breadbasket'.)

Take a look at bikers on any college campus and you'll see most of them toting their books and belongings in a light-weight backpack.

Keep an eye on them once they've dismounted and then look closely

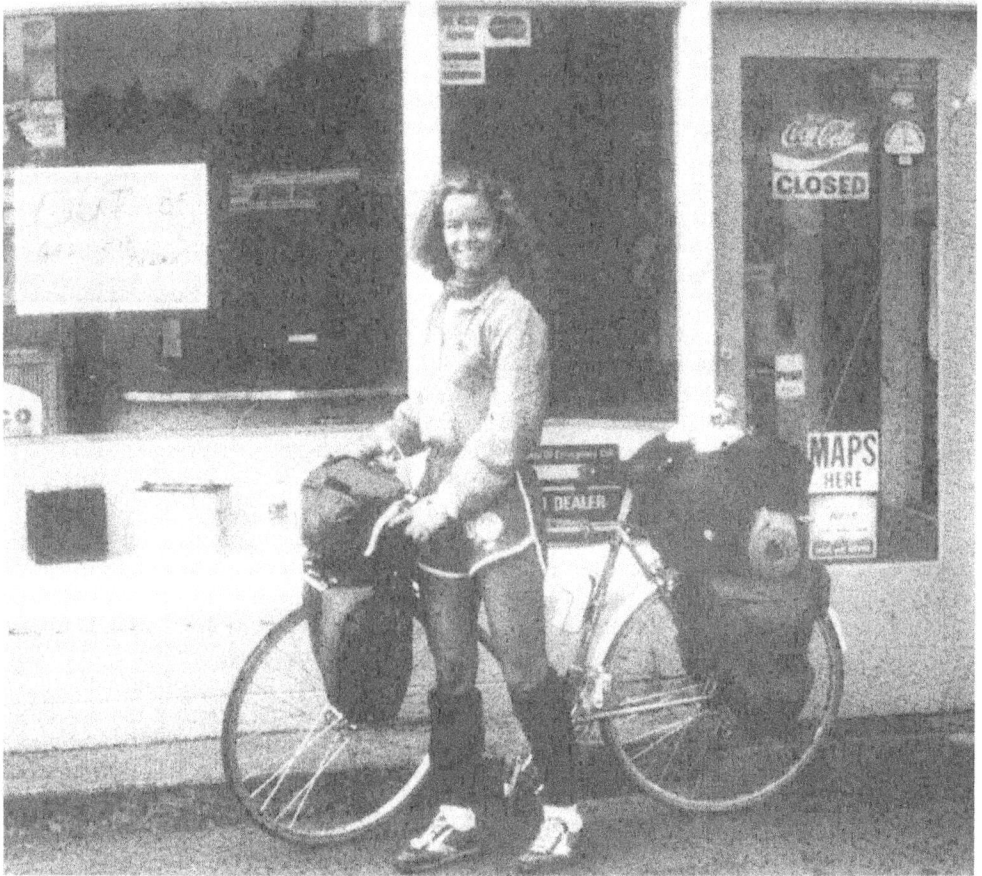

when they remove the pack you'll probably see a large perspiration spot on the person's back. Look closer still and notice the sense of relief on the rider's face once the heavy bag of books is removed - and the odds are that the rider doesn't have rain gear or tools stowed away, for their added weight probably caused them to be discarded after the first ride. Backpacks are simply not the way to carry gear on a bike. I've already mentioned the 1,700 mile ride to Canada when I was sixteen. Well, I had all my sixty pounds of gear on my back, plus a small sleeping bag on the rear carrier. That painful lesson is still present on my neck in the form of a small scar which came from innumerable turns of my head while watching for traffic. The point is, for commuting or touring, don't take a backpack.

With that option dropped, what is left? There are large capacity waist-packs, but again the weight is on you, and not the bike where it should be. Wherever the weight is carried the rider must push it forward with body strength if the weight is on the back or waist and hips then the rider must both support it and push it about. Thus I discard the waist-pack as well. And now we can discuss the real solution to carrying the commuting necessities - in a bag attached in some manner to a rack extending over the front or rear wheel. I'll discuss the various kinds of racks first, then the bags and their attachment systems.

You will recall the discussion of bike frames in Chapter One, where I spoke of the expense involved in obtaining both strength and light weight at the same time. This is also true with racks (often called 'luggage racks' or 'carriers' in catalogues). If you are dropping cars from your life and will use your bike for commuting, hauling groceries and touring, I suggest a rack which costs about twenty dollars, and which will last you a lifetime. In fact, I strongly recommend a front and rear rack - a lot of money out of the pocket but well worth the $40 for good service over that many years. (Compare that to the cost of a relatively inexpensive tune-up for your car - which might last eight to ten months.] My wife and I are both equipped with Blackburn racks front and rear; extremely strong, only 24 ounces combined weight, and almost no side-to-side sway even with heavy loads (available in most bike shops and all bike catalogues). Cycle Pro has come out with a "high quality Japanese rack. . . very similar to the original Blackburn. ..." This rack costs five dollars less, but I have to admit that I've never owned one or ridden with anyone who has. I didn't begin with a Blackburn rack, nor did I use one on my world ride in '74. For that trek I used the same inexpensive Pletchscher rack I had used for twelve years, and which yet sits unharmed in my basement. Heavier, with a good deal of lateral sway under large loads, it is a rack with the added features of a spring-type clamp for holding small items, and a cost of less than half that of the Blackburn. Naturally, good products produce imitators, and many companies have manufactured facsimiles. While any of these brands are probably sufficient for commuting loads, you should be careful not to demand too much of them on tour. Look at them closely before you buy, study the sway allowed by the long vertical support arms. And don't let a salesman hurry you along in the choice, for he won't be there on the lonely back-country road when it breaks. (A tip on mounting any kind of rack - use a bolt which threads into the rack 'eye' above the axle, not a bolt considerably smaller in diameter than the eye itself. Such a situation puts enormous strain on the bolt shank, and a breakdown is inevitable.)

Once you have chosen your rack the bag itself remains, and which kind you finally choose will depend upon highly specific needs which you alone can determine. I will tell you all that I carry for commuting;

you will add to or detract from this according to your situation, and thus choose the size of the bag you'll need. So let me present the options.

One of the most inexpensive ways to go for commuting alone is a Pletchscher rack and a nylon or canvas backpack secured to the rack by shock cords. This method is especially attractive for those who normally ride wearing the pack, for it only involves purchasing the rack for $8 or so, and two shock cords for 50 cents each. However, if more money is available to you I would move up a step by buying a bag better designed for hiking - and this can be a specially made pannier or simply a satchel of a shape more easily adaptable to bike racks.

Let me first assume you are in this all the way - and you want bags for both in-town use and cross-country use. You will commute with one bag of the set, add another if you're carrying additional books or going shopping, or add all with weight in them if you're training for tour. Once you have decided to acquire a full set of bags the next decision is which to buy. Luckily for you. almost any set you choose is better than those Wayne and I struggled with in '74. They mount more easily, wear well, and repel water and dirt far better than old ones. Let's look at some of the bags.

We'll begin with the brand Bops and I purchased in early '76 and still use - Eclipse. This company is "America's # 1 volume dealer," as their advertisements read, and there are several reasons for their success. A good pannier must be easy to attach and remove from the bike, must be constructed of a durable material, and have enough compartments to keep belongings separated on a long tour. Eclipseu-

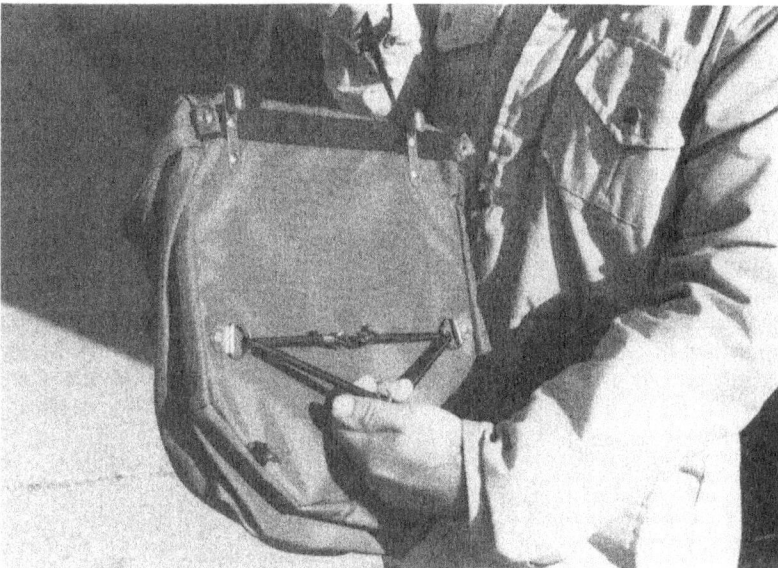

tilizes a side-mount system for attachment, with a small rod sewn onto the back of the bag sliding into the groove of the mounting plate. This mounting plate fits unto any kind of rack, and costs $6. Two nylon snap fittings sit on either side of the mounting plate, and correspond to the nylon straps at the top of the bags. Therefore, when the panniers are slipped into the plate groove they are held securely in several places - by the eight inch rod on the back of the bag, by the nylon snaps at the bag top, and also at the bottom by a metal rod which passes through a webbing sewn onto the bag. This last feature keeps the panniers close to the wheel when leaning into a curve.

This is the attachment system for the front or rear panniers (Bops and I carry four apiece on cross-country rides), and the time it takes to slip a set on the bike is about thirty seconds. The same time is required to attach the handlebar bag - a real beauty used by some of my friends as their constant companion commuting bag. The Eclipse Professional handlebar pack has eight separate pockets, adding up to a total volume of 610 cubic inches, a clear map case to allow navigation without getting off the bike, and a shoulder strap for use as a handbag while walking. It is made of a very durable Cordura material. The all-important item of suspension is where this Eclipse has excelled until the other manufacturers copied the use of a light-weight steel support frame, elasticized tension straps extending from the bottom of the pack to the fork eye, and Velcro fasteners to keep the bag secured to the frame. The cost of this bag is high - $50 - but Bops and I have used our packs for five long years and they give no indication of desiring retirement. I must say, however, that one of the metal tabs on the zipper broke off two years ago. I sent it to Eclipse requesting repair, which was granted free of charge. Try that with Detroit.

Before we leave Eclipse I must say another word of explanation concerning why Bops and I still use this company's bags. Several years ago the rear panniers came with a small fiberglass rod enclosed in cordura webbing in place of the current plastic (polypropylene) rod. The fabric covering the old rod frayed with time, and I wrote a letter to the company suggesting a modification. What I received was not only free repair of my panniers, but a phone call from the company's vice-president thanking me for my interest. With this kind of customer interest it is easy to see why Eclipse sells a huge volume of panniers.

I have described the attachment system of the panniers, but not the other features - which will be useful when I discuss other brands of bags. Bops and I tour with a Professional handlebar pack, two Transcontinental panniers in the rear, and two smaller old-style Eclipse panniers up front, similar to the present Nomad Commuter bags. The rear panniers (Transcontinental) carry the majority of our gear, and are well-designed to do so. Made of the same durable material as the handlebar pack, each pannier has six individual compartments, 2200 cubic inches total volume, are wedge-shaped to stay out of the way of the rider's foot when pedalling, and are equipped with built-in handles f6r easy transport while off the bike. For 4 1/2 years my wife and I did all of our grocery shopping using these five bags on each bike. Then, six months ago, I bought a byKart, a two-wheeled basket which attaches to the rear of the bike, and can carry loads up to 200 pounds. Though I didn't have grocery shopping in mind when I purchased it, we now use the byKart in place of the panniers for such trips. I'll discuss various kinds of carts later, but for now you should realize that a full set of panniers will work just fine for groceries.

As with all things, prices on panniers have risen considerably since '75, and the Transcontinental bags now run $105 for the pair. The Nomad Commuter panniers, with only one large pocket for a volume of 1150 cubic inches for the pair, cost $30. Eclipse puts out other kinds of bags which you may find suitable, as well as a special rack with a built-in mounting plate for the bags, and pannier rain-covers to protect the contents fully from the elements.

Perhaps the second most popular brand of panniers is Kirtland. They differ from Eclipse primarily in shape and suspension; Kirtland panniers have two hooks at the top rear of the bag, which snap into place over the rack. A heavy-duty spring hook on the bottom holds the bag next to the bike when cornering, and prevents the pannier from sliding forward or backward. I like this suspension system for its ease and for the lack of a special mounting plate. Also, the Eclipse nylon snaps on my bags gave out after a year, and rather than send them in for repair I now use a shockcord to keep them in place; the Kirtland spring-hook takes the place of the Eclipse snaps and probably lasts longer. The largest Kirtland panniers are the G/T Elite, with six pockets in addition to the main compartment, for a total volume of 2400 cubic inches. The price is $88.50. Kirtland's handlebar bag is a whopping $69, but does have 70 cubic inches additional volume. Kirtland bags come in navy blue, red, and bright yellow; Eclipse in bright orange, scarlet red, and medium blue. Finally, when you are comparing bags you'll see some, like Eclipse made of coarse-weave Cordura, and others like Kirtland and some new Eclipse bags made of fine-weave and slicker feeling Cordura nylon. Personally, I like the look of the coarse-weave. Kirtland, however, contends that the tight-weave fabric (fine-weave) holds its waterproofing qualities better.

Several pannier companies, including Kirtland, now offer bags made with "millions of retro-reflective microspheres." This makes your panniers appear as huge reflectors to drivers up to 600 feet away. Naturally, the cost is greater, but you might consider it if you'll be doing a great deal of night riding.

Are these prices scaring you? Remember that I am discussing purchasing a full set of bags with the idea of using one of them as your daily commuting bag. Alternatives to these expensive pannier sets will be discussed shortly, when I deal with bags good for short hauls or weekend rides, but not long tours. Before that, however, I should mention that Eclipse and Kirtland do not have the bike bag field to themselves. Again the tremendous competition in the bike world works to hold down prices somewhat while encouraging constant improvement, and new imitators of old favorites. In this last category comes the impressive Bikecology Class I bike packs, large-volume and well-constructed bags which cost about 25 to 40% less than the two leaders already discussed. Other popular names of manufacturers are Bellwether, Connondale, Kangaroo, and BikeWare. Check them all out before you buy, but I would suggest that you not buy any pannier which attaches with a web belt system winding through the rack top. This takes forever to put on and take off, which means an increase in the number of times you'll decide to leave the bag on your bike when going in a store or restaurant. Do this once too often and you'll lose your bag and all its contents. Wayne and I had such panniers on our world ride (they were the best we could find in '74), and I still have memories of numbed fingers working fruitlessly to disengage the web buckle in a cold rain. Stay with either the slide-on or clip-on suspension systems and you'll be happy.

Now to a couple of bags for the commuter or short tripper, large enough to carry tools and rainwear, and maybe some books and a jacket. None of these bags are specifically designed for hiking, and therefore must be attached to your luggage rack with a shock cord and some ingenuity. My first choice for the teacher, student, lawyer or reading layman is the JanSport Legal Eagle ($27.50). The Eastern Mountain Sports catalogue describes it as "Big enough to hold books, briefs, papers, plus clean shirt, emergency rations in case the jury stays out all night. Fits under plane seat." An outside pocket is divided into sections which could house tools in one side, raingear in the other - leaving the large main compartment for day-to-day loads.

While the bag just mentioned is the perfect 'soft' attache case, my choice for a single bag, if I expected such loads as those necessary to a college student during final exams, would be the Eclipse "Mini-Explorer." The bag's 1800 cubic inches are divided into five separate compartments. It can be carried like a gym bag, worn over the shoulder with an optional strap, and the 2000 pound-test nylon wrap-around

handles are also "designed and sized to permit carrying comfortably on your back. ..." The Mini-Explorer meets all airline "Carry-on" requirements, and costs $45. (EMS and Lickton's Cycle
City.)

A warning about using a single pannier to carry your belongings -Bops and I used to ride with only one loaded pannier in the rear. for it was all we needed around town to carry commuting gear. I noticed, after a couple months, that my rear wheel needed truing (spoke adjustment to align the rim). This is why I have suggested that you use your handlebar bag as a single commuting bag, or one of the Legal Eagle or Mini-Explorer types - for with all these the weight rests squarely over the wheel.

We have been a long time discussing bike bags, but aside from the machine itself, your bag is the most active part of pedalling equipment. Tools are used once or twice a month, raingear a bit more often perhaps, but your commuting bag will be with you, on and off your bike, for every day of the year. At the end of this chapter I'll review all the items I carry while commuting, but after your first year of living with a bike, your own list will be highly personalized and will go far in producing that heady independence you'll get from being a 'self-contained' unit on the road.

Bicycle Carts

As enamored as I am with the new panniers on the market, I must admit that on occasion, my wife and I have had to transport something which would not fit into any bag, or ride safely strapped onto the front or rear luggage racks. I recall the first summer in Salt Lake, when we knew no one, and needed lumber to build shelves in the closet of our apartment. We didn't need enough to justify renting a car or truck - just six thin pieces eight feet long. Granted, we could have ridden the bus, or just walked, but the problem was a challenge. Putting a few extra shock cords into a bike bag, we pedalled the five miles to the lumber yard, tied the boards on to the bikes so they extended just a foot or so from the front and rear racks, and pushed the bikes home effortlessly. (This is kid-stuff compared to Asia, where per-bike loads of 600 pounds were hauled over the Ho Chi Minh Trail for years, and where General Yamashita's Japanese soldiers with weapons and full combat gear rode the Malay Peninsula to its tip - and the defeat of the British at Singapore in '41.)

For such times as buying small lots of lumber, bringing shrubs home from the nursery, or taking the wash to the laundromat. Bops and I decided after 4 1/2 years to buy a bike cart. I wrote to the various manufacturers of carts, and found two main types - one for carrying children or light loads, and one designed for heavy-duty use of loads

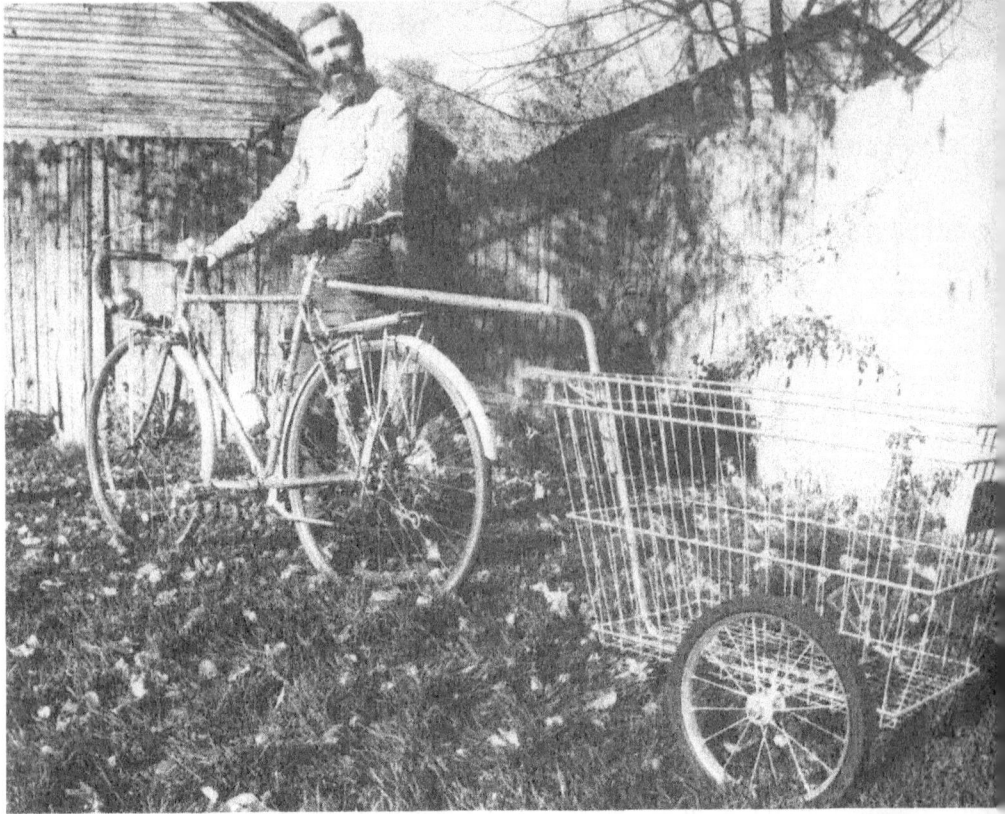

up to 200 pounds. In the first category is the Burley Bike Trailer, and the Cannondale Bugger, among others. The Bugger lists for about $190, and the child sits facing away from the rider, with a full view of the world behind. This wide view can sometimes be a detriment, however. I recall a conversation with a young father touring along the Washington coast, pulling his child in a Bugger. The first day out all was fine - until they hit a busy stretch of highway. The father said his three-year-old became strangely quiet during one long uphill climb, even failing to answer his questions. He found the reason why when he turned to look at the child, and saw him staring, frozen, at a huge tractor trailer grinding up the hill behind them only a car-length away. (One non-cart child carrier I like, while we're on the subject, is the Troxel Highback - Bike Warehouse, $25.40. It is well made, light, and sturdy attachment is to seatpost and stays with quick-release knobs. A spoke-guard keeps the child from putting his foot in the wheel.)

My purpose in buying a cart was to haul heavy or large loads, not children, and so I chose the byKart. A substantial price increase in the last year has taken the cost to about $165, including a special three-way hitch and extension bar, allowing even long loads like ladders to be hauled. Unlike the Bugger and Burley carts, the byKart has small 13" diameter wheels, which are good for heavy loads but do not guard against tipping over as successfully as the other models. I have noticed that the only times Bops and I have had the byKart tip over was when it was empty or carrying almost no weight, and that even then - when empty - it would not tip if we exercised a bit of caution in choosing our route. (When the byKart did tip over the three-way hitch kept the cart from affecting the bike, and we merely stopped and set it aright.) Children can be carried in the byKart, though they resemble gerbils in a cage due to the high wire mesh on all four sides. But if I planned to transport a child often or for long distances I would opt for a large-tire, definitely no-tip model. (Addresses in appendix.)

By the way, pulling a heavy load with a bike is surprisingly easy. I used to have images of Egyptians dragging limestone blocks to the Pyramids whenever I thought of hauling loads, but with the byKart design, a full 200 pounds adds only 15 pounds weight at the bike seatpost. The wheels mount on ballbearings, the tires are semi-pneumatic to insure against flats, and a heavy-duty steel axle supports the cart and its cargo. With my panniers, luggage racks and byKart, there are few things aside from my rolltop desk which I can't carry by bike.

We have now dealt with the commuting subjects of foul weather gear, protection from the cold, durable riding clothes, and bike bags and carts, all in this chapter designed to keep you comfortable on your bike no matter the weather or what you may have to carry. In the next chapter I'll treat the subjects of safety, first by looking at road hazards, and then by dealing with a topic I hope you won't personally experience - safety from people who might wish to do you harm. Well, you have your bike, your bags, and determination. Now let's hit the road.

3. Safety

Before we roll down the driveway and into traffic there is one main point I would like to make - the cardinal rule for pedallers who would prefer to remain with the living: *Remember you are no longer a motorist, so stop thinking like a motorist!* Let me emphasize this point with a short list of the differences between a motorist and a biker.

1. You aren't seen on a bike - drivers look for other drivers, not bikes, and plenty of times they even miss seeing the *car* they run into. Even in good weather and with non-refracting safety glass, an occasional glare off a car hood can blind a driver. For that matter, an entire automobile can perch in a motorist's 'blind-spot' behind, and even up front a quick glance can come at the time when the biker is hidden behind the thin metal strip between windshield and side window. Sound impossible? Next time you're driving test it out, and you'll see how even a narrow obstruction close to the eye can blot out large objects in the distance. (I value my occasional moments behind the wheel, for it reminds me how easy it really is to miss a biker, even when I'm looking for one. Again - the importance of the orange safety flag.)

2. You aren't feared - all motorists know the pecking order on the road - tractor-trailers, city buses, pickups, vans. Continentals and

Cadillacs, family sedans, VW's, and motor scooters in descending order. And then, at *last* comes the bicycle. Don't press your luck. You've heard about defensive driving; it really makes sense on a bike. Especially since a simple fender bender will be *his* fender, but *your* head.

3. Your presence is objected to • I know it doesn't make sense. If you were in a car you'd be taking up an entire lane, or switching lanes without signalling, plus polluting the air and contending with other drivers for gasoline supplies. But here you are inoffensively pedalling along two feet from the curb, requiring a driver only to pause momentarily and check for on-corning traffic before he swings around you. But are motorists grateful? Not on your life. It's their road, and they want you off.

I admit that some bikers antagonize motorists by riding double and taking up a full lane, or not starting off quickly from an intersection, and thereby endangering the last driver's chance of making it through the light. Some bikers also ride crazily, meandering down the street and convincing the driver that they'll swerve out in front of him for sure as he tries to pass. But even without these justifications many motorists will object to the biker, perhaps for the same reason joggers get hassled - a momentary wave of envy and self-reproach when the driver sees an obviously healthy and happy person running or pedalling along. Whatever the reason for enmity, the wise bike commuter will choose side streets and tactics designed to keep the driver, when at all possible without losing one's honor, happy.

4. You haven't the speed to avoid accidents - on a bike you can't gun the engine and scoot out of a tight spot. But travelling at such a comparatively slow speed you won't be entering many of these situations. And, once you are really at home on your machine, your increased maneuverability can assist you when accidents loom near.

5. You do not have a land all to yourself -your territory is the narrow strip of curb-side road where road-debris collects, sewer drains exist (the bars ingeniously run parallel to the curb and are just wide enough for a bike tire), cars park and drivers' doors open into you.

6. You may be a dog lover, but - don't expect that nice-looking mutt sunning himself on the front lawn to let such an enjoyable target as you pedal by without at least a chase. Usually they won't bite, but if you aren't thinking you'll swerve out to avoid the hound and be swallowed by the jaws of a Buick. I'll deal with dog attack, and proper counter-attack measures in the section on 'personal safety'.

Keeping these points in mind, let's now go for a typical city ride to work. We'll pretend it's your maiden voyage, and I'll try to guide you through the intersections and past the cars.

The Maiden Voyage

Alright, we're ready to head out. The sun is shining this morning for your first voyage to work on your bike, but resting in your commuter handlebar bag is the rain gear, medical supplies, and tools to keep you rolling no matter what. Ah - what confidence this fact gives you. (I know I haven't told you which tools or how many band-aids yet -just be patient.) Your orange safety flag flops lazily in the breeze as you straddle your bike and prepare to mount up. A quick look about to assure yourself that you really want to do this - the thoughts which propelled you to the bike shop two weeks ago float back. Then comes the chilling and bothersome thought which also has been hovering about for weeks - 'What if I don't make it?'

But it's too late. Your wife and kids are at the window to wave goodbye. Your wife's look inspires confidence; your kids' looks are sarcastic. You recall them asking, laughingly, how you planned to make it up that last big hill. . . .

You give a half-hearted smile and slip your right foot into the toeclip. Slowly, you revolve the pedal backward until you reach the 2 o'clock position, your left foot still set firmly on the ground. All systems are go -one small step for man, one giant step for society. Down you push on the right pedal, lifting yourself easily upon the saddle all in one clean stroke. As you roll along the driveway you look down to your left pedal (soon you'll do this without looking, but for now it's easier to see it). The toe of your left shoe catches the rat-trap lip of the pedal and flips it right-side up; at this moment you slide your foot into the toeclip. Success!

As you approach the street you give a quick glance to either side for cars, bikes, pedestrians. It's clear. You turn onto the street, and as you near a string of parked cars you remember to glance at the driver's side. One of the cars has a built-in headset, and it is difficult to see if a driver is present, possibly to open a door into you. Thus you glance into your rearview mirror, or turn your head quickly to see if a car is behind you. If not, you are free to move a car door's length farther into the lane; if a car is there you stay where you are, coasting so as not to gain speed, listening carefully for the sound of an opening door, and with hands on the brake hoods in case you have to stop. (This sounds awfully bothersome, but let me promise you'll find it second nature in no time. Hearing is a biker's most important safety tool after sight, and you'll soon learn to distinguish all sorts of road sounds.) You should also watch for the tell-tale movement of the driver's left shoulder slightly downward when reaching for the door handle, then quickly upward to unlatch it.

In such a situation as approaching a parked car with a driver behind the wheel, and with another car passing you on your left, you have only your brakes and lungs to protect you. If you are too close to the car to stop when the driver opens his door and you can't swerve around him due to traffic, you'll have to yell. And I don't mean some wimpy shout. I mean a full-volume blood-curdling bellow. Don't hesitate. If that door catches you as you pass it will knock you into traffic. If you hit it after it opens you'll crumple your front wheel and fly over the door onto the street. You'll be late for work, the nurse who treats you will wonder what a grown man was doing on a bike anyway, and your friends will laugh at you. So a lot rests on you being able to get that driver to keep from opening that door all the way.

My wife and I differ on this point. (My view first.) Few of us, aside from junior high school teachers and parents of more than two kids, really know how loud our yell can be. I've laid this on many drivers and never failed to halt the car door in mid-swing. The driver doesn't know what has happened, but he does freeze momentarily, and in that moment you are past him. (I make it a habit to wave thankfully once I'm past, for the usual driver reaction to his fear from the yell, and his humiliation at being forced to recognize the very existence of a non-motorized vehicle, is to chase you with his car and run over you.)

Now, Bopsy's method is more sophisticated. She doesn't say a word, but merely touches her handlebar-mounted Super Sound Bike Horn. (Bike Warehouse, $4.50 - mounting bracket, $1.50 - replacement Canisters, $4.50 for two, 100 blasts per can.) This compressed air canister then lets out an ear-piercing screech that causes seismograph needles to jump. She says it stops them every time, but I think if I were the motorist I'd leap from the car at the sound of the horn, thinking some fiend was in my back seat. I suppose I can't argue with success, but my method is cheaper, always works (the air horns don't work at temperatures below 20 degrees F.), and doesn't scare me along with the driver.

Alright, we're clear of the parked cars for a moment, and you're coming up on your first intersection. By the way, you are travelling with the traffic, right? I'm just checking, for I see a lot of bikers riding against it. I was hit once doing just that. Anyway, no cars are behind you as you reach a normal residential intersection - with no stop or yield sign. As you near it you see no cars approaching in the opposite direction, cars which could at any second decide to make a left-hand turn into or over you. Now you check side-to-side traffic. First you look to your left, then your right, then your left again. Why? Because you cross that portion of the cross street first which is travelled by cars coming from your left. Again, keep your ears open, and make use of your peripheral vision. And for heaven's sake don't commute with sunglasses which have those side-shields on them - they reduce your side-vision to nil.

You ride another block, conscious of how easy it is to propel your weight with the new gearing, compared to the old balloon-tire models of your childhood. As you pedal you realize the sun is rising behind you, and think of the difficulty on-coming drivers will have seeing anything, much less a bike. Your small two lane street has the stop sign at the intersection you are approaching; the busier four lane cross-street has none. How to cross? Basically, you'll do it in the same manner. But you have twice the data to assimilate, and you remember to gear down (into a 'lower' gear - easier to pedal) so as to be able to pedal quickly if need be. Also. think of the fact that if it is true that you have twice as much to worry about at this street, imagine the motorist -who has all this and more, for he is traveling at 40 mph and is wondering when you on the bike over there are planning to pedal out across his path. Just choose your time, and move across.

After a while your street becomes four lanes also, and when you first pull up to the stoplight your indecision as to where you should be is natural. Right turns on red may save a great deal of gasoline, but they do make it dangerous for pedestrians and bikers. Nearly every time I want to walk across some busy downtown street there sits a two ton automobile stretched across the land, edging out to make its right turn. And on my bike it's just as bad. Some drivers will look past me, or maybe through me, and pull out even though I have a green light and they've got a red. But back to you at the intersection of four lane streets. You want to continue straight on your route, so where should you be? By rights you should be allowed to take your place in the right lane, the cars behind you which wish to make a right should wait patiently for the light to change to proceed. But, alas, man behind the wheel is not mankind naked. He might be four feet tall and drive around sitting on an orange crate to see out the windshield, but he's got metal all around him and a hundred horse-power at his right foot. So chances are he won't sit patiently idling behind you if he wants to make a right turn. He'll blast you with his horn, or try to squeeze the nose of his beast between you and the curb. He knows it won't fit there, and is counting on you to edge to the left a bit to let him get by. Therefore, to keep the world happy, and right turn motorists from rolling over me, I stand straddling my bike at a point left of center of the right lane. (This is of course if I'm at the head of traffic in my lane. If not, and the driver ahead of me is planning to go straight, then I'm okay because the other drivers are mad at him.) This position allows the cars behind me to turn right as they wish. If I stood next to the curb in the right lane the cars turning right would have to come very close to me as they passed. As soon as the light turns green, but after my own glance left and right tells me it's clear, I pedal from left of center in the lane, back to my usual position near the curb, so cars in my own lane can pass me. One mile from home now, and all is fine. The saddle is a bit uncomfortable, but you've been told to expect this at first, and are assured it will go away after the first week of consistent use. It's time to make a right turn to head uptown, and you pause to catch your breath and recall the route you planned with your topographical map the night before.

Planning the Route with Topographical Maps

Service station maps are fine for motorists, but bike commuters should have a map which tells differences of elevation as well as distance. I use the 7.5 Minute Series topo maps, for they provide extremely detailed information. Distances are measured at a scale of roughly 2% inch to the mile, and schools, churches, parks, shopping centers, hospitals, and other major buildings are drawn in and labeled. This is helpful in determining the amount of traffic a particular route might carry, and what hours the traffic would be heaviest. For example, I never route myself past a school between 7 and 8:30 a.m., or 3 to 4:30 p.m. Shopping centers are fine before 9 a.m., but I avoid them like the plague after that. Drivers travel the wrong way in lanes, throw open doors without looking, leave carts everywhere, and keep dogs hiding in the back seat to roar at you from the window as you ride by. Hospitals are fine to pass, except for the emergency entrance and exit, and churches are great at all times except for the Sabbath. And whatever you do never ride past a church when it's letting out. I've seen motorists who minutes before listened to sermons on fellowship with meek smiles on their faces cut one another off and roll over bikers to be the first one out of the church lot.

A detailed road classification is also provided by topos. Different colorings or markings indicate the categories of Heavy-duty, Medium-duty, Light-duty, Unimproved dirt roads, and Interstate, U.S. and State highways. The map symbols include everything from footbridges and overpasses to dams and canals. Various shadings indicate swamps, wooded marshes, vineyards, orchards and more. And if your daily ride to work takes you past a glacier, your topo map will show you the best way around it.

Concerning differences in elevation (always of immense importance to pedallers), 'contour' lines are placed on the map and a specific 'contour interval' is designated. The maps I use for navigating Salt Lake have a contour interval of 40 feet; the vertical difference between the contour lines is therefore 40 feet. If my first choice for a route when I sit down to my topo map has several of these lines within a few inches

I know I'll be doing some climbing. The numbers on the contour lines (feet above sea level) will tell me if I'm climbing steadily or traversing rolling hills. And, if the lines are bunched together (as is sometimes the case in Salt Lake and San Francisco and other very hilly areas), the biker knows to take a rope and alpine climbing axe with him, or choose another route.

The 7.5 Minute Series is set up on a scale of 1:24,000; one inch represents 2,000 feet (approximately 2%' to the mile). Thus, the entire map covers a small area - between 49 and 71 square miles. Less detailed topo maps which cover larger areas are the 15 Minute Series. These have a scale of 1:62,500, with one inch representing about one mile. Weekend trips can be planned with the U.S. 1:250,000 Series, with one inch representing about four miles, and State base maps at scales of 1:500,000 and 1:1,000,000 are available for all the Continental States. (Alaska and Hawaii are covered by state maps at other scales.)

Many public and institutional libraries have these maps, but if you prefer to own yours you should call the nearest Geological Survey office and ask if they sell topo maps. (This is a Federal office, so look under United States Government in your telephone white pages.) If they don't sell them they'll probably know a nearby commercial dealer who does, but private dealers sell at their own prices. The best way to obtain them if you can't find a nearby USGS office is to order them from one of the two following addresses:

(for maps of "areas east of the Mississippi River, including Minnesota, Puerto Rico and the Virgin Islands of the United States,")
  Branch of Distribution
  U.S. Geological Survey
  1200 South Eads Street
  Arlington, Virginia 22202
(for maps of "areas west of the Mississippi River, including Alaska, Hawaii, Louisiana, American Samoa, and Guam.")
  Branch of Distributing
  U.S. Geological Survey
  Federal Center
  Denver, Colorado 80225

You should first write to request an Index to the topographic maps of your area. and the prices. (When we moved to Salt Lake I bought the four 7.5 Minute Series maps necessary to cover our commuting distances, at $ 1.25 apiece.) While you're requesting your Index ask for the free booklet "Topographic Maps," which explains the use of these maps in 27 clearly written and easily understood pages.

Okay, you've had enough of a rest. As I recall, we left off with you about to make a right turn toward the business district of town. All the savvy of an animal in the bush is necessary to negotiate a business district without winding up as a hood ornament, so keep your wits about you. You are already riding as far to the right of the street as is possible, so making your right turn won't be any trouble. Just keep an eye and ear out for cars which also wish to turn right, but can't seem to afford the ten extra seconds required to follow you through the turn. Sometimes a car will hurry along to a position parallel with the rider, then make the turn as the bike does, only cutting the cor-ner sharply and thereby restricting the biker's maneuverability. If you don't know your route well, an unexpected sewer drain could be waiting for your front wheel, or if you aren't looking ahead properly you might round the corner and have to dodge a pedestrian in the crosswalk, or a hopeful bus rider leaning out into the street looking for his ride and muttering despondently about public transportation. (This may appear to be a good time to stop and suggest cycling to him, but it isn't. People want only instant solutions to periods of frustration, not suggestions for future times. If the fellow is less than a half hour late for work he'll probably stand sullenly nodding his head, hoping someone will run over you. If he's already later than that he'll prob-ably take your suggestion and your bike, and leave you on the curb with his bus pass.) Even if you do know your route, and know that a sewer drain is not present, a broken bottle might be. If so you'll have to swerve to avoid it, and if you've made your right turn at the same time as a car, your room to swerve is gone. Moral: only make right turns when cars aren't saddled up next to you in your lane.

Another mile without any trouble, and now you are downtown. You've been careful at each intersection to watch for on-corning cars wishing to make a left-hand turn across your path. At stoplights you've geared low so as to take off fast when the light changes. At the wide and busy intersection where there should be a stoplight but isn't, you let two cars next to you (heading in the same direction) run interfer-ence across the street so you could pedal alongside safely. But now you have to make your first left-hand turn at a light, and you aren't sure how to go about it.

There are three methods of making left turns on a bike, and I use all of them depending upon traffic conditions. Let's assume you are turning left at a busy intersection downtown which has no separate left-turn lane, but does have a left turn arrow. Unlike right turns, you must begin planning a half block ahead for a left in heavy traf-fic. If the cars are moving slowly, and if you have the orange safety flag mounted on your bike so you can be seen, take advantage of a break in the traffic to move into the left lane. When doing this I try to make eye contact with the driver behind me, I signal my intentions with my left arm, and move sharply across the lane. Now I am wheeling toward the intersection in the left lane, and my major concern is to keep the car behind me from rolling over me if I make it to the intersection after the left turn arrow turns to solid green. Again, if a car ahead of me is also waiting to turn then I'm okay, but if I am the vehicle holding up traffic I must be sure to be seen first by all drivers, and next to get out of the middle of the intersection as soon as possible. Thus the first method of making left-hand turns on a bike is the same as a car - but with the condition that you vacate this left lane immediately, and exercise extreme caution in moving there from your usual right curb-side haven of security. In addition, when making a left turn in this manner you should not turn into the left lane of the next street, as of course we are instructed as drivers. Instead, if no cars are present you should fade into the right hand lane, while listening for the occasional driver who will gun it to get by you on the right after following your turn from the intersection.

The second and third methods are much more time-consuming but infinitely safer, and are almost a necessity in stop-and-go rush hour downtown traffic. Both involve dismounting momentarily and executing two steps - and which of the two you choose will depend upon the light when you arrive at the intersection. First, if the light is green and you haven't been fortunate enough to move into the left lane, continue across the street, hop off your cycle, and walk your left turn when the light changes. You have now reached the right-hand side of the street you wished to turn on to, and can remount.

If the light is red or amber when you approach the intersection, however, pull to the right, dismount, and cross the street you had been riding on. Then, waiting for the light to change, push your bike across-the street, mount up, and shove off. (One warning here - when pushing a bike in a crowd be careful to allow for pedal room -1 have more than once clipped a passerby in the shins.)

Your left turn is past, and now there are but a few blocks remaining in your ride. You are close to success, but a bit fearful because of the long hill you have yet to climb. Before you begin, pull over and rest yourself, and let me run a few more pointers by you. Do you feel warm? Chances are you haven't noticed this for all the attention you were paying to the road. Open up your shirt a button or two, and pull up your sleeves. Now a few more tips:

1. We all know what a 'rolling stop' is, and most of us are guilty of them occasionally. Bikers, just like motorists, do the same. When there is no cross traffic, and when a real momentary stop is made even while still in the saddle, I can't see any sense in dismount-

ing. (Should you someday be ticketed for not putting a foot on the ground at a stop sign, you might refer the judge to certain world record books which include a contest of staying balanced on a bike, with both feet in the pedals, without forward or backward movement. I can do this for several long seconds at a stretch, plenty of time for me to assess the intersection and move on - all without coming out of the toeclips, and still having a true stop.) But one thing I have seen and suggest you guard against is the tendency for a biker to fade with cross traffic at an intersection, then suddenly scoot across the street when the cars are past. This is not only illegal, but very dangerous, and is not worth the hassle saved by stopping completely at a corner. After all, what's a few seconds more or less?

2. Don't over-react to the blast of a horn. This is easy to say but difficult to follow, for the only time a loud honk won't startle you is when it is expected, and a rider can't clutter up his mind all day with this thought so as to be constantly expecting it. What a rider *can* do is condition his responses away from the natural lurching forward in the saddle and quickly pulling on the handlebars to the right. (Instead, work at changing that reaction to a gripping of the handlebars, and just the bars, *not* the brake levers.) This response keeps you from being forced into an accident, and denies the motorist that sense of satisfaction from having blasted you off the road.

3. When entering driveways or other entrances from the street, watch out for a difference in height between the street and driveway pavement level. Oftentimes there will be a V2 to 1 inch rise - just enough to jolt an unsuspecting rider, or even enough to throw him if he has not taken the driveway at a sharp angle. Because of the mere 1" or so height of the bike tire a 1 inch lip of pavement above street level can be dangerous. If your commuting route takes you along old state highways you will sometimes find a similar lip of road surface above the shoulder. I've seen more than one rider bite it when, pedalling along the shoulder, he forgot to angle his front wheel sharply to climb back on the road.

4. Always try to appeal to the driver personally - for as long as the face-off is between a car and bike you will lose. Make eye contact with the driver, use your wits to communicate your intentions, and chances are the motorist will see that communication is between humans, not unequal vehicles. This is especially important in situations where you as a biker would have the right-of-way if

you were in a car. Example: a four-way residential intersection with no stop or yield signs; as you approach you see a car coming to the intersection on your left. You are thinking he'll yield due to position, but he might assume you'll stop because you're a bike. At these times I make it evident that I'm not planning to yield by retaining my speed. However, my hands rest on the brake hoods for a speedy stop if necessary, and I glance toward the driver to indicate that I am aware of his presence but still do not intend to stop. As difficult as it may be at such times to wave thank-you, or show it with a smile that you appreciate the driver doing what he is after all supposed to do, it will help the next time this driver is in the same situation. If, on the other hand, you see commuting as your arena of gladiatorial battle against the enemy auto, and gloat at the driver as you pedal past, you'll do a great deal toward turning that motorist against bikers.

5. Be especially careful around cabs and buses. Cabbies are a queer sort who appear to believe in their charmed lives, able to drive about in today's cities without getting smashed. Due to this success they become assured their driving skills are beyond question, and because they make their living on the streets they erroneously believe they have a greater right to these streets than we. Don't bother arguing these points with cab drivers -just avoid them when possible and don't trust them to relinquish the right-of-way. Buses are not trustworthy either, but in their case the reason is less difficult to ascertain. Simply, they're bigger than everyone else, and drive like it.

Alright, you're rested, and I've had a chance to offer a few more tips on safe riding. Still straddling your machine, you have only a bit further to go. Mount up, watch the traffic, pedal evenly and slowly, inching up that last hill. Use your gears to keep from straining, so you won't be too warm when you finally make it to work. (I've noticed that most of my visible perspiring takes place once I've stopped riding, and thus I make it a point to push easily for that last mile.) Your sense of self-satisfaction is growing with every turn of the pedals as you near your destination. You are very awake and ready for work, unlike the days when you drive along in a near-stupor. And you are happy in knowing that whatever the evening brings you will already have gotten the exercise that is so often missed due to late dinners or unexpected company. With the sun and wind on your face you won't have to use your lunch break driving to the nearest downtown fad shop for a ten minute, twenty dollar tan.

And now you're in front of your destination. We'll talk about how and with what to lock your bike in the section on self-protection, so for now just dismount and wait for your friends to come out and congratulate you. (Be prepared for the kidding, and be good-natured about it, for if you are, you might convert them to bikes in time.) Finally, don't forget the money you've saved. Be happy with yourself. You deserve it.

(Allow me to mention here that all the non-bikers think a ride to work requires a shower afterward. That's bunk. For three seasons of the year 'layering' your clothes will permit you to jump off the mount and begin your day; in summer I like to run cold water through a washcloth, apply this to my face and chest, then buff dry and put on a clean undershirt. This routing takes 4 minutes, requires only a sink, and is very refreshing.)

I've used the phrase "fair-weather" riders earlier in describing 95% of cyclists, and to be perfectly candid I can't view them without a certain amount of disdain. These riders remind me of the people I see clogging city parks in summer, but who are absent for the other seasons of the year. As I ride past I hear the blare of the radios drowning out any birdsong or solace one might otherwise have found in this wedge of nature amidst the buildings. I suppose what gets me is the sense of loss I feel when I think of what they are missing - the same loss that 'fair weather' riders experience by not meeting the rain and snow and cold on their bikes. Perhaps if more riders knew how to keep warm and dry in the elements, and how to ride safely throughout the year they would give it a shot. I've already told you how to dress properly. In the next few pages I'll describe the riding techniques I use in snow and rain and even on ice, and the times when I would suggest you hop a bus or hail a cab. After all, with saving so much money by cycling you can afford a cab when you need it.

Riding Techniques for Rain, Snow, and Ice

Most of you reading this probably live in climates which produce more rain than snow, so we'll begin with drizzles, move on to downpours, next snowstorms, and finally icy streets.

Rain: To all the aforementioned precautions for dry streets, add the following.

1. Even during a light drizzle a motorist's visibilty is reduced - and greatly reduced for many due to poor windshield wiper blades. Don't hastily assume you've been seen.

2. Motorists, who for the most part seem to think they'll shrivel up like the wicked witch if they get wet, do not expect bikers to be on the road when it's raining. Not that they look for us at any other time, but during inclement weather they hardly believe our presence even when they do see us.

3. If drivers often have poor wipers up front, it is at least preferable to the almost total lack of vision they have to the sides and rear. Don't follow a slow car too closely.

4. Imagine yourself behind the wheel, talking to a passenger, listening to the radio, hearing the raindrops on the car roof and windows, and the wiper blades as they swish back and forth. And now you are the biker outside trying to communicate with the driver by yelling something to him. My point is, don't count on the driver seeing or hearing you in the rain.

5. Automobile accident statistics indicate that drivers greatly overestimate their ability to stop, especially on wet roads. Even during a light drizzle a car tire can 'hydroplane' if the motorist doesn't know to pump his brakes to break through the film of water on top the road surface. Thus a tire is actually sliding along on this water film, greatly increasing the braking distance. Let's face it - the driver can live through his error in judgement about his ability to stop in time - but you can't.

6. Not only is the motorist's sight, hearing, and ability to stop his vehicle reduced during rain, but the cyclist's difficulties in all these areas are increased as well. Rainstorms are difficult for eyeglass wearers - my wife has found her contact lenses invaluable for rain-riding. When wearing a rainhood be sure to tie the drawstring so as to secure the hood to your head - this way it will turn when you do. Otherwise you'll look to the side for traffic and see only the inside of your hood.

7. Keep your hands on the handlebars at all times in the rain. This will help to compensate for the inability to view the road for a good distance with a single glance, as you do when streets are dry.

8. Although I do not use them myself (due to the cost), I have acquaintances who swear to the stopping ability of Mathauser brake pads even when they are wet. For myself I trust my senses to warn me away from dangerous situations, and my ability to leave my saddle quickly if necessary. This attitude of letting my bike have the accident whilst I bail out may sound callous, but it has kept my skull somewhat structurally sound. (Set of 4 Mathauser brake pads in metal shoes -Bikecology. $8.)

9. Avoid riding in the very center of any lane on wet streets for this is where oil drippings from innumerable passing cars accumulate; especially on black-top roads water droplets will rest on this oil and create a slippery spot.

10. You should always cross railroad and streetcar tracks at right angles - that is, with your front tire perpendicular to the direction of the tracks. Especially in wet weather this must be done, for wet tracks are unbelievably difficult to cross without slipping if you are careless on the approach. Sit squarely over your frame as you pass, and have your bike perfectly straight while you are on the tracks.

11. When cornering, do not lean as much as you would normally. Make wide turns so as to allow the bike to remain more upright - thus lessening the chance of having your mount slip out from under you.

12. Avoid riding directly through deep puddles, if possible. Such pools can hide broken glass and other objects which will damage your tires.

13. Finally, it helps to know your route well for rain-riding. Potholes on blacktop surfaces sometimes fill up in a hand rain and look much like the surrounding pavement. Also, you will know where to expect sewer gratings, increased traffic, et cetera.

So much for riding in the rain. Our next topic, snow-riding, may seem ridiculous at first. But, again, if you are careful you'll not hurt yourself, and will instead open up that final season to experience -winter. You might reply that you experience it already, during snowball fights with the kids or while skating or skiing. Think for a moment, though, how many times you really do these things from November through March. Most people appear to dread winter, thinking of it as a time of difficulties - walkways to shovel and cars not starting, and increased driving time to work and home. And what a shame. They have lost that childhood excitement of seeing huge flakes blanket the earth, or romping in the fluff or just listening to the stillness which envelops the city following a storm. In my mind I see two images of the same person separated by twenty years, first a boy of ten, his face a single huge smile as his eyes take in the falling snow outside the classroom window; next a man of thirty, hunched over papers at his desk then despairing as he glances up to see the snow fall.

You might contend that this is natural, for the boy is hoping school will be closed, while the man knows his work will go on. And this may partially be the case. But the boy won't detest the snow when he finds school will convene the following day. He still loves it, for it is something enjoyable. To the man, however, it is merely bothersome.

My point is that by getting outside and into the snow, by riding carefully through side streets and viewing a landscape changed in an hour, the storm ceases to be a bother and instead becomes an experience. For most of us, challenge has left our everyday life, adversity gone the way of the sweatshops, perseverance now a quality exercised most often in simply living an urban life of few challenges and many frustrations, seldom washed away by the purgative of fresh experience. For me, riding through the snow to get to work on time is that challenge, that goal, that experience. Drivers think it's crazy to see a biker in the fluff. But what they don't see, hidden beneath the goggles and muffler and ice-encrusted beard, are my smiles.

Snow: All of the suggestions above apply, as both rain and snow create wet streets. However, snow requires some additional precautions.

1. Always keep the bike as upright as possible. This is especially difficult as we turn corners and maneuver about on dry streets by merely shifting our weight and leaning over; do this in snow and you'll be on the ground in no time.

2. Pedal evenly. A good rider does this normally, but even a single powerful stroke can unbalance a rider in some snow conditions. I try to imagine myself cranking along in slow motion when I ride in snow, for this reduced cyclic rate makes it easier for me to remain balanced.

3. Don't ride at full speed. As with rain puddles, in snow you can't see what obstacles may be in your path. Long before winter I have my snow route chosen - which may be different from the normal commuting route due to less traffic, cleared streets, or any number of reasons. Be sure you know your snow route *before* the first storm -you don't want to ride into sewer gratings or potholes lurking beneath the flakes.

4. Learn the 'tripod' technique (my own invention). When going downhill in snow, brakes alone will not be enough to slow you sufficiently for safe riding. Therefore, on downhill runs and at any other time when a spot is especially slippery, lift yourself off the saddle, sit on the top tube, and put one foot on the road. You won't be able to pedal in this position, but then you won't need to as you are trying to slow down and regain your balance. Naturally, sitting on the top tube is uncomfortable, but you won't be there long. (One of the boys in my high school bike club solved this problem by mounting a very narrow second saddle directly to the tube. Ah - ingenuity!)

5. Don't use your rear brakes in snow (or ice, sand, or gravel, for that matter). I have found that rear brakes cause a fishtailing of the back wheel in bad areas, and can cause a spill. Whereas slamming on the front brakes at such times will likewise throw you out of the saddle, easing on the front brake will allow you to feel through the handlebars any attempt of the front wheel to slide left or right. Once this is felt you can compensate through the handlebars; a slide in the rear wheel is much more difficult to counter.

6. Avoid automobile tracks through snow if the car tires have not reached *through the* snow to pavement. Usually car tires merely pack down the snow, and make for very slippery riding. Bike tires, on the other hand, cut through the flakes with their narrow profiles and often will make good contact with the road.

7. Because of the width and poor traction of automobile tires, watch out for cars sliding your way. Often the panicked driver will slam on his brakes when he begins a slide, which locks the tires and skids them merrily along on top the snow. If you live in an area which receives only one or two snowstorms a year, watch out. Drivers in such areas never seem to learn, or perhaps just fail to remember, how to drive on white streets. Again, your snow route should be relatively free of traffic. And if this can't be done then get up a bit earlier and miss the rush. (Besides - there's a certain thrill to being the first one to put a narrow groove through the snow.)

8. Fresh snow is much easier to negotiate than that which has had a chance to crust or freeze over during the night. Therefore, be even more on your guard the second day. Sometimes I am forced to ride in the car tracks on such days due to the frozen ruts turning into driveways or curb-side parking slots. But be careful when you follow these tracks, for getting out of them requires an acrobat's skill.

9. Some cities salt their streets in winter; others use cinders or sand. With the last two, and especially with sand, a biker really has his work cut out for him in not slipping. Just be careful, pedal evenly, and for heaven's sake go slow.

Ice: Even the thought is chilling. Yes, bikes can be pedalled across ice, but then, some people can swallow swords, too. To begin with, I don't ride after ice storms. But plenty of times I've hit patches of ice between relatively easy-to-traverse snowfields, and have therefore found ways to stay on my bike across these spots.

1. Pedal at quarter-speed, if you *must* pedal to get across. I try to coast across ice patches, and immediately go to tripod position when I see ice (it's less of a fall from the top tube than from the saddle!)

2. Never apply brakes on ice unless you want to spill. If you wish to stop go to tripod and drag a foot. If it's an emergency you'll have to gear it to stop fast, so know beforehand how to take a bike down. When I want my bike to stop with me I pull the right side of the handlebar toward me, while throwing my rear weight to the left. This causes the bike to swing in an arc toward the right, and to slide downward with me to the ground. You might think going down on the left (non-derailleur) side would be preferable to save your changers. But doing so would pull you to the middle of the road; a right-hand take-down pushes you toward the curb. Besides, I've never damaged a derailleur in this way, for my leg is always beneath it! People often ask experience. For most of us, me if a rider can come out of the toeclips, and the answer is yes. In fact. even though spills are much more prevalent in winter, and therefore one might think in best to be out of the clips, I find that they prevent accidents. For example, the tripod would be dangerous without a clip to hold your foot in place on the pedal.

3. The worst time to be on ice is when you aren't expecting it. This usually happens with what is called 'black' ice - generally a very thin veneer over blacktop or other dark road surface.

4. Finally, there are small strips of tread studs for bike tires, and I have often thought training wheels front and back would be a great assist on ice. But it is easier, and wiser, I believe, to admit that some days are not meant for travel on two wheels. (The thought imparts a proper respect for nature and a healthy humility at the same time.) Though I've not been stopped one day in the last five years, I have paid for my impudence with some dandy spills, and ended up walking by bike a half-block to assess the damage to my joints. I can recall times in college, however, when ice storms put me on foot for most of the trip. And though it is difficult to admit it, the sudden switch from cycling to walking was as pleasant as the move from car to bike. Sure it took a long time to get anywhere on such days, but isn't it right that some days be unique, troublesome, time-consuming, and memorable?

Besides, there are other alternatives. Cross-country skiing is a relatively simple means of travelling across the flakes, though one wouldn't guess it by watching me flounder about. Buses, once they arrive, are special places to be on winter storm days. When I board and see the huddled bodies peering out the windows I think of ancient thick-brown hominids in a cave entrance, their startled expressions lit up occasionally by the flash of lightning which drove them there. And in the war, while mortars searched for us at night, we edged closer together for that same camaraderie which modern American life does its best to forget. We live with the horrible isolation of a 'civilized' world, in which man can travel to and from work, and from coast to coast, without interacting with fellow man except to stop on red and proceed on green. Moving to bikes can't change all that. But the subtle differences of thought which come outside the automobile world, and the slowing down of life's pace, can help.

Personal Safety - Self Defense

At the end of a long, dry day of headwinds in Montana we reached a parched outpost of three houses and a cafe, clumped together in a valley which no doubt the early settlers had hoped would blossom and become a town. Our mode of travel brought on the usual conversation, and after a while I turned the questioning around. I asked them how it felt to live so far away from cities, and one sundrenched face smiled as it replied, "Well, now, we kinda like it. Part of it's the quiet, I guess. But mostly it's knowing that here, in our valley, we have to count on ourselves for everything."

I've thought about that comment often, and use it here to introduce a very unhappy topic, one which I hope you'll never have to employ -self-defense. My opinion on this subject is similar to the rather incongruous fact of peaceful nations possessing great armies and navies. Simply, weakness appears to invite attack from the demented few. Bikers, who appear vulnerable to motorists, must be able to respond to such hassles personally, and not merely hope a policeman will be near. In other words, even in a city of millions, we cyclists must be able to count on ourselves.

Now, please don't misunderstand. I'm not talking about packing around a 44 magnum and emptying it into anyone who yells at you from a car window. (This pistol is far too heavy for bikers - try the snub-nosed 38 with drilled-out handle instead ... ha - just kidding.) What I am suggesting is a rational appraisal of the *chance* that someone might cause trouble, and a preparation for that moment so as to appear ready and willing and capable of self-defense - an attitude which, when perceived, will help to deter any escalation.

There are some cases where you may have to fend against a carload of jerks out to take advantage of a lone rider, or where you may meet up with a malicious character who intends robbery or worse. Again, the commuter will probably never run into such a situation. Most of us never see our antagonists; they yell their words as they are speeding by, throw their firecrackers or squirt at us with fire extinguishers, all because they can race off to distant safety with impunity. (That is, unless we catch their license plate number, which allows for - and demands for the good of fellow-riders - an extension of the battle on fairer grounds.) But let's assume two punks in a car have decided to rough you up a bit, and step through your alternatives. Chances are if you have not a good bit of training in the martial arts you would have a rough time against two people. Therefore, to even the odds somewhat, I suggest that you carry two excellent weapons on your bike.

The first weapon is merely a water bottle, but filled with straight ammonia. To give yourself confidence that this is an effective deterrent to crime try taking a good sniff of it yourself - and then imagine catching a strong spray of the stuff in your eyes, nose and mouth when you are least expecting it. (Some people may fear that use of such a chemical is illegal in their city, as is the case with mace in some areas. You could call the police and ask, I suppose. But I wouldn't bother with it. Until the state can guarantee my personal safety while on the road, I'll remain equipped as I feel necessary. I'd prefer the later legal hassle to any physical injury.) If two guys hassle you, you have several options; pretend you are bored with the whole idea and remove your bottle from its holder while the goons approach, then spray the closer of the two and, while he is choking proceed to teach the second fellow a lesson in manners; second option - spray both fellows and then beat on them a little; third choice - spray both and continue pedalling. The problem with this last option is that in fifteen minutes when their tears have washed the ammonia from their eyes, they will probably be looking to run over you. Therefore, I suggest a minor modification of the above. No matter which of the options you prefer, consider ending the bout by removing the car keys from the ignition and tossing them into a field in the country, or down a sewer if in town. More than likely anyone stupid enough to hassle another human just for the pleasure of hurting him will not have a second set of keys nearby.

The second weapon which should be on every bicycle is the safety flag. I prefer the thin, rather rigid single-piece fiberglass flag, mounted on the axle of my front wheel. If trouble looms and I think a simple swat across the face will make someone think twice, I merely reach out to the flag, invert my hand so as to be swatting the base of the rod and not the flag top when I swing it, and remove the flag from its holder. The sting of such a rod is great, and is very difficult to guard against as it can be moved so quickly through the air that it is actually invisible - like the tip of a bull whip.

The last weapon which I carry is one which I suggest only to those who have had specific training in its use, and such self-possession in times of crisis that one would not go over-board with it and cause someone's death. I am referring to the knife. Please let me reassuringly interject that in fifteen years of riding I have never had to use a blade, and have had to draw it only once. Perhaps I would never have begun carrying it had it not been for my daily route through a ghetto of St. Louis, where, on occasion, I had bottles and rocks pitched at me. Had I not been trained to use a knife in the Army I would not have carried it even then - for a blade is usually the final escalation of an argument before grievous bodily injury results. There are ways to hold and use a knife where only flesh wounds will result; but put this weapon in the hands of a novice and a simple jab toward the chest can make you a killer. At the worst you'll be sent to jail for defending yourself too strenuously. At the best you'll still have a person's life on your conscience, and carry the memory to your grave. If your route requires it, and if you know what you are doing with a blade and won't hurt someone unnecessarily or have it taken from you and given back in your ribs, then I suggest the Buck Esquire 501 locking-blade pocket knife ($23). It is excellent in construction, is made of stainless steel which can stand up to all seasons without corrosion, and the lock-blade feature keeps the cutting edge from folding down upon your fingers. But, most importantly, I have found that with several drops of Liquid Wrench or other light-grade oil, and with much working of the blade back and forth, the Esquire can be out of the pocket and open for use almost as fast as a switch-blade. This is accomplished by holding the knife with the second joints of the fingers, and, with the fingertips, pushing the blade out from its resting place in the handle a half-inch or so. Next a quick flick of the wrist causes the weight of the blade to fall the rest of the way out of the handle, until it clicks into place for use. The clicking sound is also good, for it brings attention to the knife, and if any light is present the stainless steel will glint its reflection. Your opponent will think you are carrying a switch-blade. You want him to think this, and you want him to know you can use it and will if you are forced. All this is necessary so that you will not have hurt or be hurt.

My middle road on weapons for the biker is merely to be ready, to have the option of self-defense. Don't get carried away with apprehension or let self-defense turn to offense, but merely take care of yourself. The world needs all the good people, and especially all the bikers, that it can get.

At the risk of appearing sexist to some who do not allow the physical differences between men and women, I will now suggest a particular tactic on self-defense for females. Whereas my wife does carry weapons with which to protect herself, she also carries an item which, when sounded, might well halt the attack by scaring the assailant. This item is the Super Sound compressed air horn I spoke of earlier (Bike Warehouse, $4.25). It should be blasted as loudly as possible *before* an expected attacker is close by. An early blast should make the thug realize that his escape is the best way to avoid an awakened neighborhood. However, if you wait until the person is almost upon you his choice will probably be to lunge and knock your hand from the horn.

A second item along this line is the police whistle worn around the neck on a braid, or attached in some manner to the handlebars with an elastic cord which can be stretched easily to the mouth. (I don't prefer this method, however, because it will either be stolen off your bike within a month, or become a hassle in itself if you take it off each time you leave your bike. Such items added to the bike frame, but not secured against theft, become those things either left at home - "Well, I'm only going a mile to the store!" - or left on the bike with the logic of "Who's going to steal that?!" This is why I have all my necessities in the single bag I ride with, except for one water bottle of ammonia. When I stop both bag and bottle go inside with me, and I needn't fret about thieves.) As mentioned earlier, the compressed air horn will not work at temperatures below 20 degrees F., so a police whistle is a good stand-by for cold nights. Also, don't forget what I said about the power of the human lungs; a blood-curdling scream should go far toward bringing assistance.

Of course, women, just as men, cannot afford to rely upon changing an attacker's mind or recruiting help. My wife works the second shift at a hospital several miles from our house, and therefore rides home in the dark every night. She has the air horn on her handlebars for easy reach, but also carries the water bottle of ammonia, and a very small canister of Mace with a pen-like clip for her pocket (available in sporting goods or department stores for $6 on up). This tiny canister possesses a powerful spray, can be hidden in the hand, and should be concealed from the view of the assailant until he is within sure range. This requires a degree of self-composure which only a great deal of forethought on this subject can provide. As distasteful as it is, think through the incident slowly and in detail, imagine your fears and reactions, and practice extracting the Mace from your pocket until it becomes effortless. Then, when you are fully prepared for something which will probably never happen, you can ride with confidence.

And now to the subject of dogs, one of the greatest headaches for bikers until one learns to deal with them effectively. I have, in the last fifteen years, tried almost every imaginable tactic with canines. And the trustworthy ammonia in the water bottle is the best find yet. With this I have stopped huge mutts in their tracks, and my aim is now so good that I can drench a hound's snout without ever getting it into his eyes. (As with people, ammonia will wash out of the animal's eyes in a very short period of time, but just a good whiff of the stuff is sufficient to halt a dog, and there's no reason to be malicious. Besides, I always fear a momentarily blinded dog will wander into traffic and be hit.) Since there is nothing permanent about this technique, except for the memory of the dousing in the dog's mind, I find this superior to the method I am forced to employ on tours, when all my water bottles must unfortunately carry only water. This second tactic is the use of the safety flag as a whip. However, the rider must be careful not to hit the dog's eyes with the flag tip, and also not to unbalance himself in the saddle when leaning over to strike.

I once read an account of a rider who said he went through four frame-mounted bicycle pumps beating off dog attacks in Baja California. With the cost of pumps this rider would have been ahead to carry a stack of round steaks to throw to the animals when they gave chase. Pumps as weapons are a poor choice (though I did brandish one once, in a poor section of Cairo when a throng of teenagers surrounded my friend and refused to let him pass). Tire pumps are too short, too light and malleable, and the handle slides away from the base whenever it is swung downward.

Other methods include yelling loudly at the dog in a commanding tone (seldom works), shooting a Mace-like spray at the mutt called •Half (Bike Warehouse, $2.40), and if you can believe it, beaning the hound with rocks carried in the front handlebar bag (as a friend in

Salt Lake does). I have even read a suggestion in a hiking magazine that it was *our* fault the dogs attacked in the first place. The reasoning went something like this - 'dogs are fearful of people looming high above them, therefore bikers bring on the assault by sitting so tall in the saddle. The solution is to dismount when the dog nears, bending over so as to lower your stature, while talking to the animal in a soothing tone.' I must admit I often enjoy Sunday cyclists and their ideas, but not when the advice is dangerous. To begin with, I'd never get anywhere on my bike if I stopped every time some mutt charged, except perhaps to the hospital when this silly tactic didn't work and I was half-eaten by a wolfhound. And to my mind this entire method is wrong in attitude, for it requires the biker, the innocent party, to mollify the animal which is in the wrong. Granted, because it is an animal we cannot make a moral judgement of its action, but I can sure do so with the owner who by law in most cities must have his dog on leash or otherwise under control when outside.

I recall an instance only a few months ago which occurred on a residential street near my house. Riding home from work in the early evening I was startled by the appearance of a huge German shepherd bounding out toward me from his yard. His gait wasn't that of a dog on attack, but nonetheless I glanced quickly to my rear, saw that it was clear for me to swerve to my left, and reached for my ammonia. At that moment I noticed a young man sitting on the porch of the house from which the shepherd had run, and I yelled to him. "Hey! Call in your dog!"

"Oh," he replied, disdainfully, "he won't bother you." I saw red instantly, wheeled the bike around and charged up his driveway.

"Dammit, he's already bothering me!" I yelled. "What if a car had hit me when I swerved to get away?"

My reaction had shocked the fellow, who, as most people, expected a person on a bicycle to react in a simple, accepting, childlike manner. In Europe bikers are hassled much less by motorists, not because Europeans are innately nicer to one another, but because bikes are not viewed as kid's toys. Therefore adults on bicycles are still adults, and are treated with greater respect. Once I pulled into the man's driveway and demanded responsibility for letting his dog wander about I was an adult in his mind. As such my words were weighed, and the fellow answered, rising from his chair and approaching me. He apologized, saying he hadn't thought that a biker might swerve into a car to get away from his dog, and said it all so honestly that I was immediately embarrassed for *my* actions. I stumbled out a few words of understanding, and pedalled off.

Finally, self-defense on a bike is an unhappy topic to write and think about, and a disagreeable experience no matter what the result.

Ultimately, the choice to be made is who is going to be hurt, and how badly. Fail to protect yourself against the creeps in life and you may be maimed or killed; resort to prayer when a dog attacks you and you may be bitten or knocked into traffic. But, if prepared for such events, you will be in the advantageous position.

Protecting Your Investment—Locks

I can recall seeing a Western a long time ago in which a man was hung for stealing a horse. It seemed pretty severe to my young mind, for my ethical training to that point placed a horse's value far below a man's life. I couldn't understand the anger in the man with the rope - until someone stole my bike many years later. And then I prayed I would find the thief, and planned what I would do when I caught him. Luckily, I never did. The loss of the bike was terrible, especially as my financial situation was gloomy at the time. The sense of being personally assaulted by an unseen and therefore unreproachable assailant was difficult, for it allowed no chance for expiating the anger through physical or legal means. But worst of all is the memory of knowing that I could easily have done great damage to the thief had I found him, and would momentarily have felt justified in doing so. That anger, that bestial rage and desire to maim, was unpleasant to experience then, and unpleasant now to recall.

You can save yourself from those emotions by securing your bike with a good lock, and by knowing how to lock the bike properly. Twice in the last year I have winced when seeing a single wheel locked to a bike rack in the city, for I know what had happened. An unthinking cyclist had wheeled up to the rack, pushed the bike nose first into the slot, and locked the front wheel to the metal rack arm. And a minute later a thief merely flipped the quick-release lever on the front wheel, backed the remainder of the bike out of the rack, and wheeled it away. I have also seen several bikes with the frame and rear wheel securely locked to a rack, but missing the front wheel. In this case the thief gets away with less, but you are still out the $50 replacement cost of a wheel. And it needn't happen.

How have my wife and I solved the problem of bike theft, after all these years of riding through America's cities and leaving our bikes outside stores and theatres and restaurants for hours unobserved? Unfortunately, the candid answer is that we have only solved the problem for ourselves by making it difficult to steal our bikes, in comparison to the majority of cycles poorly locked and therefore obtainable with little effort. Don't be like me, who had to lose a good machine before he learned how to protect it. And don't squabble about dropping $25 for a lock, when it secures an investment of ten times that and more. The 'penny-wise, pound-foolish' adage still applies.

Now, let me describe the three main types of locks available, the best kind to use, and how to secure your bike with them.

The three types of locks are: 1) chain and lock, 2) cable and lock, and 3) shackle. The chain type is that which is usually bought at Sears and secured with a huge key or combination lock. The cable is usually a braided coil-type of many individual metal fibers banded together and encased in plastic. The advantage of these kinds are that when of sufficient length (six feet) they can thread through a bike frame, both wheels, and around a tree or telephone pole. The disadvantages, however, are so great as to totally disqualify them for use by a serious commuter. Allow me to list the problems.

1. *weight* - 5 to 10 pounds (!)

2. *bulk* - how do you carry these huge boa-constrictor size monsters? I have seen them wrapped around seat tubes, or carried in a bike bag which was wearing out quickly from the load, or even, (as my wife did once before we were married), worn around the waist and secured by a key or combination lock. (In this case Bopsy had borrowed a brother's lock for the ride downtown, forgotten the combination, and couldn't get the brother later by phone. Thus the day was spent going from store to store with a long cable and lock wrapped about her waist, while her bike sat unprotected.)

3. *ineffectiveness* - none of the cables or chains are as successful against theft as the three shackle types I'll mention later.

4. *grease pick-up* from chain - when a long chain or cable in threaded through a bike frame it often comes into contact with grease and dirt build-up. This transfers to hands when packing up the lock, and invariably then to clothes and bike bags.

In short, don't count on being happy with a cable or chain lock, and don't bank on your bike still being there when you go to retrieve it. They look impressive, so you'll be attracted to them immediately. But look around first. You'll save a lot of weight and probably your bike as well.

Several years ago a friend who owns a bike shop in St. Louis called me and said he wanted to show off some new equipment. I pedalled to his shop, expecting a new derailleur assembly or homemade frame, but found instead a hoop-shaped lock clamped tightly in a vise.

"Okay, thief," he said, "have at it." And with this he handed me a hacksaw.

I attacked the hoop and quickly heated up the blade with furious sawing, but in a few minutes had only formed the slightest groove in the metal. Astonished, I turned to Bill, who pushed a hammer my way with the words, "Whack it a few times." I did so, concentrating the blows upon the lock mechanism. No luck. Next I was handed a jeweler's screwdriver, to manipulate the lock. I tried, again to no avail.

Finally, my friend placed the jaws of a 36" bolt-cutter on the lock and invited me to give it one last try. I squeezed the handles until my face was beet-red.

"Okay," I sputtered, out of breath from the final attempt, "you win. I'll take two."

This is an honest account of the way I purchased my Citadel, one of the three shackle-type locks which *Consumer Reports* (July 1980) rates as best. The cost is $25, which entitles the owner to $200 payment from the company if the bike is stolen as a result of lock failure. The weight is 1.9 pounds, though a longer-shanked Citadel, weighing and costing a bit more is now available. *Consumer Reports* rates the Kryptonite 4 and the Magnum as equal to the Citadel, though I've not tried either of them. (Most bike shops will have these locks, and all bike catalogues.)

Now, how do you lock your bike after you have your nearly impervious Citadel? First, be sure to secure your bike to something which would be as difficult as your lock to cut through. (Example: I once knew a lady at a hospital in St. Louis who locked her bike to a small tree. Her work shift over, she returned to find that a latter-day Washington had sawed through the trunk, though he did not remain to admit the truth, or the whereabouts of her bike.) I've also seen bikes locked to cyclone fences, which take but a few seconds and a small pair of wire cutters to snip through. If it has to be a cyclone fence for you, lock around the vertical fence post support.

Once I've found my fence or rail or bike rack to secure to, I use my Citadel to lock around the frame *and* rear wheel. This of course leaves my front wheel for the taking, so I use a tiny cable and padlock to secure the wheel to the frame. My reasoning on this is that while a thief could use a bolt-cutter to steal my front wheel, he won't risk getting caught for just a wheel, while so many other bikes can be taken whole for the same amount of trouble. (My wife's reasoning on this matter is a bit different, and she carries two Citadels for real security.)

Shackle-type lock manufacturers recognize the front wheel problem, and suggest a remedy which is, I suppose, fine for the infrequent rider, but far too great a hassle for a commuter. Their suggestion is to take the front wheel off the bike, lean in against the frame, and lock it with the same Citadel which is securing the frame and rear wheel.

Unfortunately, this requires many seconds each time the bike is left, both to take off the wheel and to replace it later. And I begrudge every unnecessary effort in securing my bike. With my easily detachable commuting bike bag and two simple locks, the act of securing my bicycle is almost as quick and simple as closing and locking a car door.

Well, so much for your safety. Be careful, and good luck to you.

4. Mechanics

First off, let me say that if a picture is worth a thousand words, the experience of watching someone make repairs on a bike, before you try it alone, is worth a million easy. Secondly, ability in mechanics does not necessarily coincide with intelligence. And third, try to have the right tool for the job. I recall my amazement at the speed with which mechanics completed their tasks at the Dodge dealership I worked at long ago, dropping engines and tuning engines and swapping water pumps in a quarter the time my friends and I had required in backyards and alleys. The difference - they had just the right tool for the job. Now, when out on the road you won't be able to carry all the sophisticated machinery you'll have collected in your basement or garage, and I'll give you some tips on what will work in a pinch. But, at the beginning, you should realize it's much easier to get the job done with the correct tools; and if you don't have them, and can't afford to buy them, then go easy on yourself when simple adjustments take longer than you think they should.

What follows is a concise treatment of maintenance and repairs which commuting and touring will require, including the adjustments of handlebars, saddles, and brakes. Unless you have a keen interest and ability in mechanics you will probably never take a derailleur completely apart, and therefore do not need the information on how to do so. If, however, you decide sometime later that you would like to dismantle your components (and even try to put them back together again), I suggest *Glenn's Complete Bicycle Manual* as a guide. For me, the last 40,000 miles of riding have never required that I take a derailleur completely apart, and I hope things remain this way. I clean and lubricate my bike when deteriorating performance tells me it is necessary, but, I'm afraid, I don't do much beyond that. Besides, I've never met a compulsive bike cleaner who was a longdistance tourer or all-weather commuter as well - I think they can't bear the thought of all that dirt and grime. So, don't look for a complete mechanics guide in the following pages. All I'm giving you is everything I've needed to know in the last fifteen years on my bike.

No sooner will you get home from the shop with your beautiful new bike than an adjustment of the handlebars and saddle will be required. In fact, you should expect to be making minor adjustments for the first few days on a new machine, until it feels like part of you when you mount up.

Saddle

Recall the earlier discussion of saddle height. If it isn't correct you'll need to change it. Begin by examining the saddle and the way it is affixed. (Most things are very simple on a bike and almost self-explanatory. Whenever you have a problem, study the matter a bit before you reach for a manual; let your head try to intuit the relation-ship between parts, and next what might not be working properly. I think you'll amaze yourself at what you can figure out on your own.) You can see that a saddle can be adjusted in four ways -height, tilt, a movement forward or backward to increase or decrease the distance from the saddle nose to handlebar stem (gooseneck), and movement from side to side. Let's run through these separately.

1. Height - your saddle sits on top of the seat post, which must be raised or lowered for the adjustment we wish. Now what holds this seat post in place is the bolt which goes through the frame directly behind the post itself. The bolt head is usually round, with a small metal tip beneath it which fits a frame slot, designed to hold the bolt steady when tightening the nut on the opposite side. Usually, just loosening the nut will allow the post to move, especially after you've had the bike for a while. To get it to move you'll have to take hold of the saddle and twist it from side to side, pulling up or pushing down at the same time. (I use bike grease or petroleum jelly on my seat post to keep it from freezing or rusting in place.) Once the saddle is at the height you wish, merely tighten the seat post bolt nut, and you're done.

Where as vise grips, channel locks, or a crescent wrench will all do the job, I suggest you refrain from using the first two mentioned due to their serrated teeth, which leave unsightly hash marks on the nut. Personally, I couldn't care less about the aesthetic beauty of my seat bolt nut, as long as it does the job. But since you'll always have a 6" crescent wrench in your bike bag, you may as well use the correct tool. And a word or caution when using crescents - if you don't buy a good wrench, and if you don't snug the sliding jaw right up to a nut or bolt head, there is a good chance that you'll 'round' the corners. Do this a few times and you'll have real trouble getting a hold on the nut at all. In my basement I have a full set of open and box-end metric tools, and so if home, I use one of these to insure an even greater fit seat post nut. But, on the road, the crescent is my choice.

2. Tilt - each rider finds a particular slant of the saddle preferable to him, if of course he knows that such a choice is available. To produce this angle you will need, on most saddles, two wrenches; any of the three mentioned above are acceptable, though I prefer a vise grips and a 6" crescent. The saddle underside has two long metal bars which run nearly the length of the seat, and which are wider toward the rear, narrower toward the front or nose of the saddle. Attached to these bars is a double clamp with a hole in the center for the seatpost, and a single metal bar threaded on both ends. This bar runs through the two clamps and has a nut on either end; tighten the nut and the clamps tighten upon the long metal bars beneath the seat, while also narrowing the center hole and thereby securing the saddle to the seat post.

While the saddle is on the bike, place one wrench on one clamp nut, holding it fast. (This is why I prefer the vise grips, for it holds by itself and frees my hand.) With the second wrench loosen the second clamp nut until it moves freely; then, apply force to the saddle rear or nose to move it into place. Finally, tighten the clamp nut securely. If you look closely at the clamps you will notice grooves or serrated edges on the clamp faces, to help hold the saddle in place. When you tighten the clamp nuts make sure the grooves are matched properly.

3. Forward and backward movement - this adjustment facilitates riders who, while taking the same size bike due to leg length, have arms of different length. Much earlier I mentioned the availability of different sized handlebar stems for this purpose, and also the technique I employ of tilting the handlebars up a bit to allow for easy reach of the brake hoods. The saddle is also designed to aid in this fitting.

To slide the nut forward or backward, merely loosen the clamp nuts as in '2' above, position the seat where you wish, and tighten the nuts again.

4. Side-to-side movement - the nose of the saddle should point directly forward over the bicycle top tube, but will sometimes be cocked to one side or the other if the seat post bolt has worked loose. To straighten this you should, as in * 1' above, loosen the seat post bolt nut, position the saddle correctly, and tighten.

Note: Some bicycles with center-pull brakes have a metal bracket attached to the seat post bolt, and movement of the nut on this bolt can tighten the brake cable by tilting the bracket up. I usually place the flat side of a crescent wrench across the metal bracket and gently push it back into position.

Note: Some fancy saddles have attachment systems other than the clamp-type just described. One such model has two bolts pointing downward from beneath the saddle, therefore making it quite difficult to reach the bolt head with a regular wrench. Special wrenches are available for this purpose, which are bent like a flattened S, but I would never commute or tour with the extra weight.

Handlebars and Headsets

Problems with handlebars usually fall into one of the following categories:

1. loose bars
2. loose brake lever
3. need for new bar tape
4. bars difficult to turn from side to side
5. need to raise or lower bars. Don't forget we are talking about the 'drop-bars' of Chapter One.

1. Loose bars - handlebars can be loose in two ways; they can slip upward or downward, and they can slip from side to side while your wheel is still heading straight down the road. With bars slipping up or down the remedy is to tighten the handlebar binder bolt, located in the middle of the bar. at the end of the stem. Most bikes require a small crescent wrench for this adjustment, but some have an alien head. (Alien wrenches of the correct size only should be used;

sometimes a smaller-size alien can be made to turn the bolt by using the wrench at an angle. However, this wears down the inside of the bolt head, and therefore should be avoided.)

Bar slippage from side to side (while the wheel remains straight) requires a tightening of the handlebar expander bolt, the head of which rests on the top of the stem or 'gooseneck'. By tightening this bolt the 'wedge nut' is pulled up inside the stem, thereby expanding the stem wall against the head tube, and locking it into place. (A second popular style of expander bolt system is the angled expander, which works in the same way.) When making this adjustment I straddle the

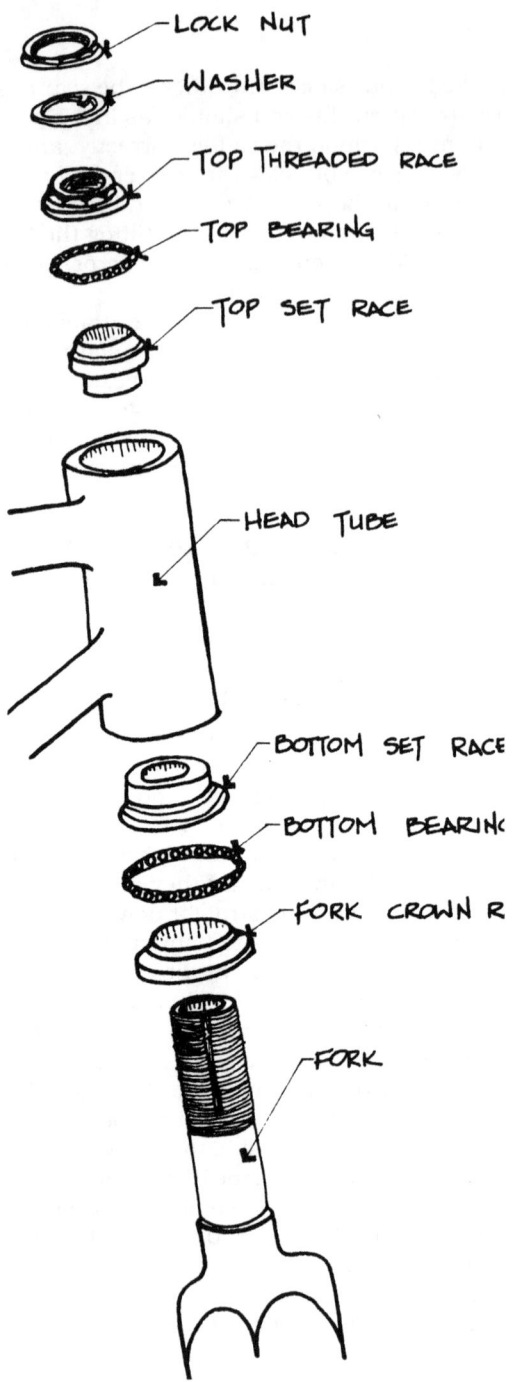

LOCK NUT

WASHER

TOP THREADED RACE

TOP BEARING

TOP SET RACE

HEAD TUBE

BOTTOM SET RACE

BOTTOM BEARING

FORK CROWN R

FORK

HEADSET

front wheel, facing the bicycle, placing my knees on either side of the fork. When I am sure I have the bar positioned properly I tighten the expander bolt.

2. Loose brake lever - if you ride a great deal with your hands on the brake hoods your brakes will, after a long while, slip downward on the bar. To remedy this you will first have to trigger your brake release (if you have one), or remove the brake cable from the brake, or remove the brake pads. (For clarification see the section on brake repair.) This is necessary so as to be able to depress the brake lever fully on the bar, thereby exposing the apparatus which holds the brake hand lever on the bar. You will see a screw-head directly behind the brake cable; this is what must be tightened to prevent further movement of the lever. If you use a long, thin-shanked screwdriver to turn the screw you won't have to remove the brake cable to make the adjustment.

3. New bar tape - handlebar tape, like all things on these beauti-fully aesthetic and efficient machines, makes the bike look complete, and performs a necessary function. That multiple function is: a) to allow for a good, fast grip on the bar, b) to absorb perspiration from the hands, and c) to cushion you from road shock. Cloth and leather tape provide for all these needs; plastic tape, however, has only its bright color going for it, and represents a Detroit inroad into hik-ing which will be stamped out once riders understand the form and function of their mounts. Tape should be added when old tape wears out; when I used cloth tape I always wound new over the old, both for greater absorption and so that I might have a thicker bar to hold with my large hands. During the last eighteen months I have used all-leather tape, which I find the best yet. I oil it just as I do my leather toe clips and straps and saddle, and it has held up beautifully. (Bike Warehouse, $6.50)

Replacing tape is not difficult, though it requires a bit of practice. I always begin at the top of the bar next to the stem, with two or three wrappings laid over one another. Next, I begin by angling across the bar, overlapping each winding with approximately one-third of the next. I do not remove the brake hand-lever or brake hood for taping, but merely wrap around it. The tricky point is ending up with the right amount of tape at the end of the bar. This tape end will be secured in place by removing the bar and plug, stuffing the tape inside, and replacing the plug securely (which often requires a sharp rap or two with a mallet or hammer or heel of the hand). There is no problem with having a good deal of extra tape left over, for you will just cut off the excess, leaving the necessary two or three inches to push into the bar and hole. (But first check your windings; tape manufactur-ers know exactly what length is required, and I have never wound up with an excess.) If you are short by a few inches, which invariably happens the first time or two, just rewind carefully, overlapping a tiny bit less each time.

4. Bars difficult to turn from side to side - this problem, though at first glance a handlebar-related difficulty, is actually the fault of the headset. The headset secures the fork to the frame but must also allow for free movement of the fork to either side. The diagram of the headset and fork will show how this dual purpose is made possible;

the top tube of the fork is threaded, and held in place in the head tube by the top threaded race (bearing cup). This race, and the fork crown race, are positioned with the top and bottom bearings to allow for rotation. In all my riding, the greatest difficulty I've had with headsets was remedied in a fifteen minute repair: first, using a large crescent (10" or greater) when home (my small channel locks on the road), I loosen the large lock nut at the top of the headset. Next I loosen the top threaded race, but only slightly, until I can see the bearings inside, but before they can leap out and hide from me on the floor. I then squirt cycle oil into the mass of bearings, very carefully allow the fork to slip down a fraction of an inch to expose the bottom bearings, and add oil there. This being done I tighten the top threaded race, then the lock nut on top, until there is no upward or downward movement within the headset, but free movement of the fork from side to side. (Your top and bottom bearings may be set inside a small metal retainer cup. If so, you stand a smaller chance of losing them; apply oil as indicated.) Now, if you drop some bearings out of the headset, and do not know if they came from the top or bottom races, you'll have to take *all* the bearings out of both, divide them in half and replace them. If you come up with an odd number of bearings, even after searching everywhere on the floor and your pants cuffs, you have probably lost one. Take a bearing to a bike shop, and buy some of the same size.

A word about bearings - whereas headsets are not usually a problem, wheel and crank bearings sometimes need replacing, and not just oil or grease. A bearing should be round and smooth on its surface. Sand and the usual road grime will tend to 'pit' bearings, and after a while will flake off a piece of the surface. If these bearings remain in your bike they will wear upon axles and races until they too will require replacement. Bearings are extremely inexpensive compared to these parts. So don't forget the axiom about an ounce of prevention.

5. Raising and lowering the bars - this procedure gives many riders fits, for they don't understand what you already know about expander bolts and wedge nuts (reread * 1' above). Usually a rider will loosen the expander bolt completely, then straddle the front wheel

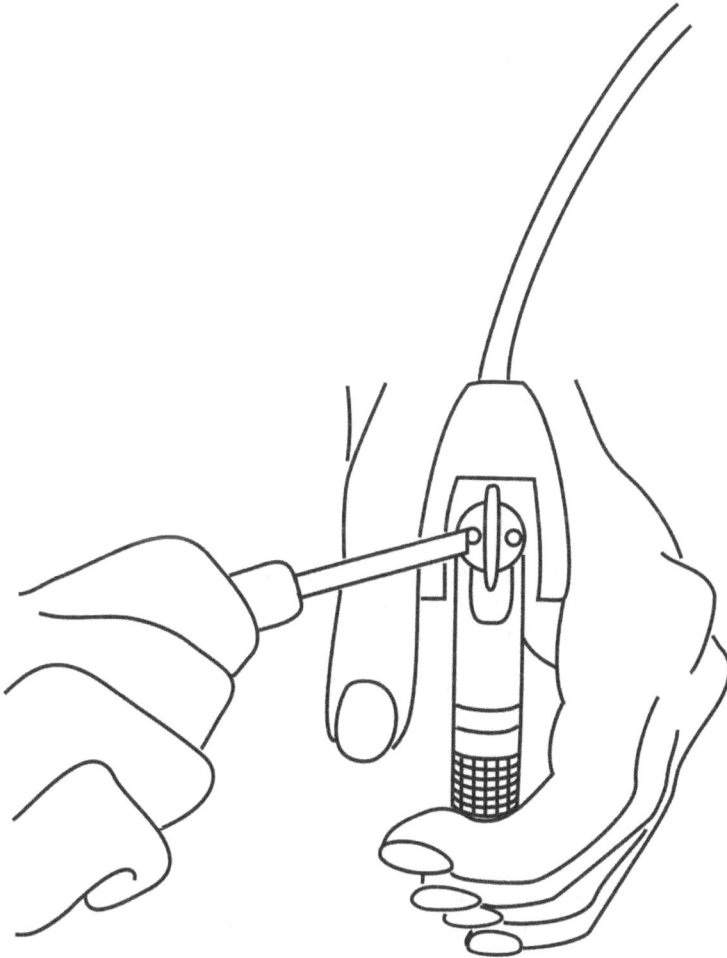

and tug at the bar for all he's worth. The problem is that the wedge nut is still frozen in place. To remedy this, the expander bolt must be rethreaded a few turns, and a sharp rap with a mallet delivered to the top of the expander bolt. This will free the wedge nut, and by turning the handlebars while pulling up or pushing down at the same time, you will be able to raise or lower your bars.

Note: always leave 2" to 2 1/2 of stem in the headset for a proper and safe grip.

Wheels
(tires, tubes, rims, spokes, axles, bearings, freewheel removal)

We'll discuss wheels in the following problem categories:

1. flats ('punctures' to the British)
2. wheel alignment
3. broken spokes
4. bearing maintenance
5. freewheel removal

1. Flats - one of the real pains in life, and a true patience-tester. Flats will never come to you when you have plenty of time to make an appointment, are out wheeling just for fun, or when you're with a pretty girl and would like to have a simple breakdown so you can have more time together. As few punctures as you'll have to deal with in life (if you are following my suggestions of good tires and PR tubes) you can count on them coming your way as you're riding toward an important job interview, or when you're already late for work. So be prepared with the necessary tools, and the experience of having gone through the motions at home at least once before. I hate facing a new mechanics problem for the first time on the road; I'm not telling you to drive a nail into your tire for practice, just go through the process of removing the wheel and breaking down the tire at home.

The tools necessary for this repair are:

a. Tire levers - small metal levers used to pry the tire bead from its seat in the rim. You only need two, but of course most manufacturers sell them in lots of three, for about $1. The levers should be steel, not aluminum (more weight, I know, but the lighter ones always bend on me), and should have a hole cut away on one side so as to hold onto the spokes. Also, if your shop or bike catalogue has levers of two different lengths choose the longer ones, for they'll be far easier to use and thereby justify the additional weight.

b. 6" crescent wrench - to remove the wheel axle nuts, unless you have quick-release wheels.

c. Tube patch kit or new tube - the patch kit costs about 50 cents, has a tube 'rougher' (to make the rubber more adhesive), glue and patches of different sizes.

A word of warning: this very simple repair can be troublesome until you've done it a few times - like learning to tie your shoe laces. So don't complicate matters by substituting screwdrivers for tire levers. Screwdrivers were designed for screws, and will only put holes in your tubes and rips in your tire if you use them in place of the correct tool. Even on the worlder in '74, when I pared every imaginable

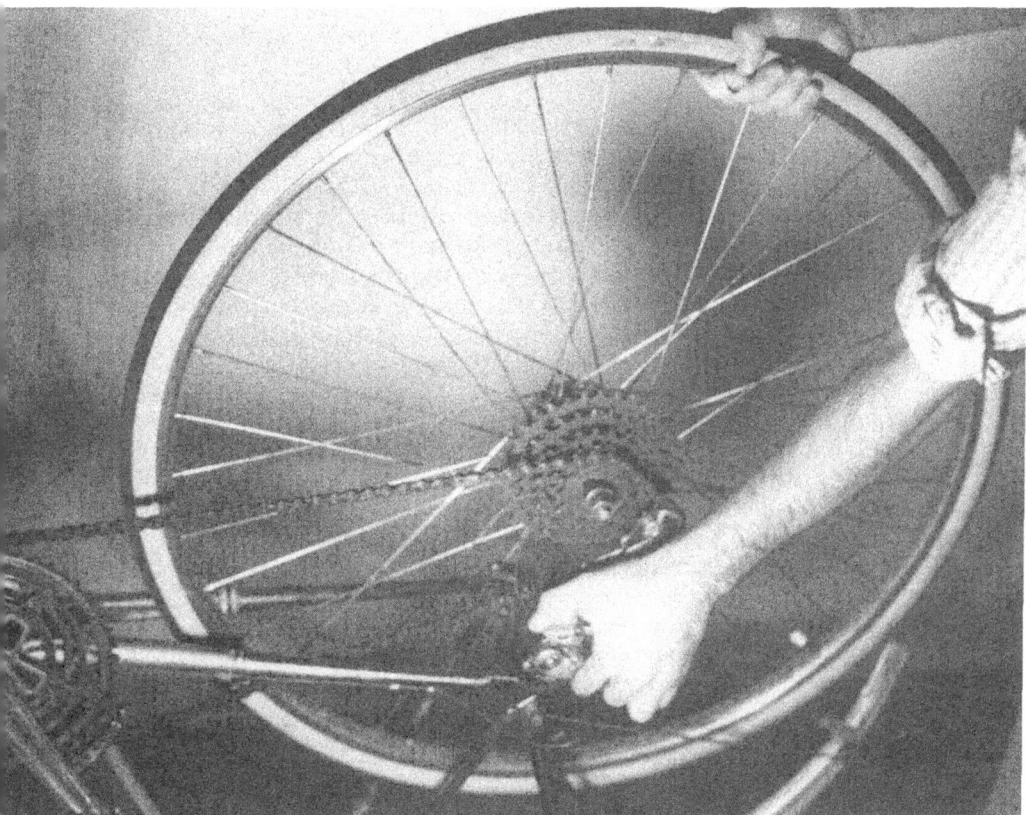

bit of weight from my touring load, I still carried tire levers. And now back to fixing a flat. (Steps 'A' through 'K')

a) You must begin by removing the wheel from the frame. Let's deal with the front wheel first, since it's considerably easier. You will recall that I spoke earlier of releasing the brakes, in the section on handlebars. This release is necessary because of the width of the tire being somewhat greater than the space between the brake pads. Most expensive brake sets have a quick-release mechanism operable with the flick of a finger. I didn't have this convenient option until a year ago, and therefore merely used a crescent wrench to take off one of the brake pads. (See section on brake repair.) Some riders prefer to remove the cable, by squeezing the two brake pads together on a centerpull brake and slipping off the cable carrier, or the barrel cable end. Whichever you prefer, once the brake pads are out of the way, you may move to the next step.

b) Release the wheel, either by tripping the quick-release on the hub, or loosening the axle nuts.

c) Pull the wheel away from the frame. This may require a degree of effort, for the fork blades are sometimes machined so as to be actually narrower than the axle. Also, study the dropouts so that you will be pulling the wheel in the correct direction.

Note: I do all this while my bike is on its back. for this is the way I do it on the road. Some riders suggest the use of a bike rack at home, and prefer to lay the bike on its side (never the derailleur side) when on the road, rather than upside down. Their reasoning is sound, for putting a bike on its back will, in time, crack the cable housing coming out of the hand brake levers. However, spoke replacement and wheel alignment require the bike to be upside down, so I merely place a couple turns of electricians' tape on the cracked housing, and forget about it.

d) If your rear tire is flat (and more than 90% of all my flats have been in back), you'll have more difficulty in removing the wheel. First, trip your quick-release brake lever or remove one brake pad. Then shift the chain into the smallest sprocket on the cluster. (It does not matter which sprocket in front holds the chain.) Next, trip your axle quick-release, or loosen the axle nuts. Holding the wheel with your right hand, reach to the rear derailleur housing with your left. and take hold of the body. Gently, pull the derailleur up and back toward yourself. This will move the chain out of the way of your small sprocket, and the wheel can be removed.

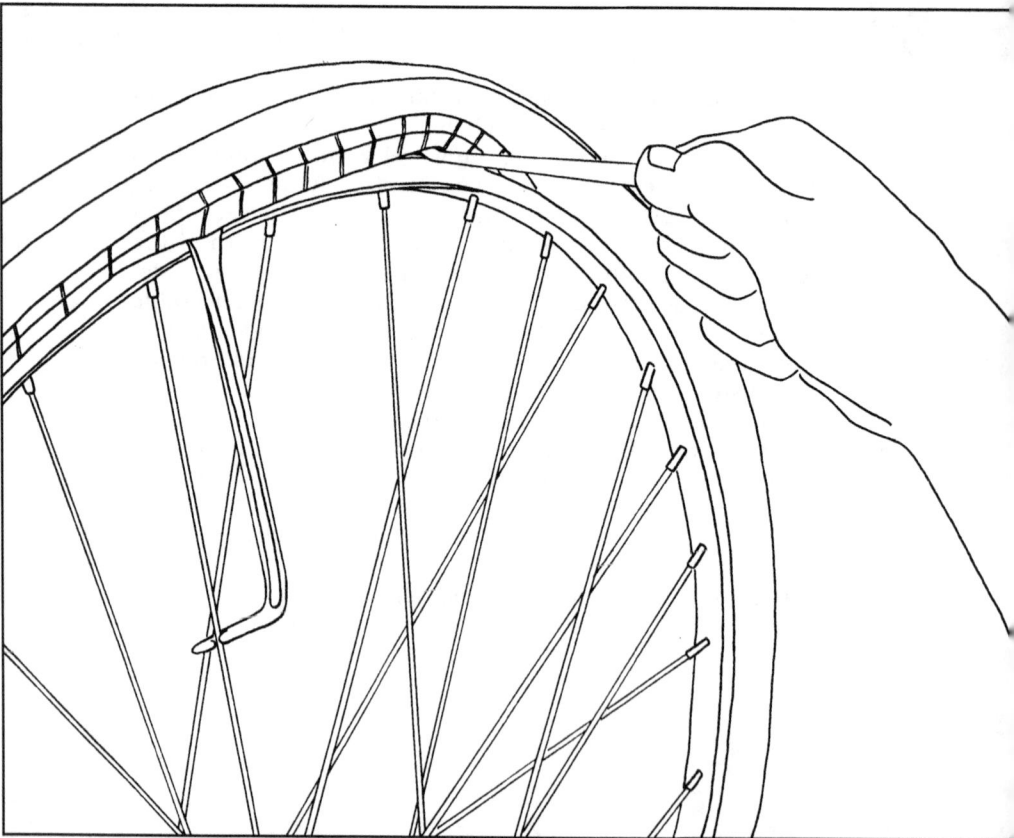

e} Remove the tire and tube from the wheel. This is accomplished with the aid of your tire spoons. Take the lesser-angled end of one tire spoon and, beveled-end up, work it underneath the tire bead about a half-inch. Now push downward on the tire lever end in your hand -that is toward the spokes. Hook the slotted side onto a spoke to hold the tire in place. (This frees both your hands for the rest of the work.) Take a second lever and, once again, work the tip underneath the tire bead, about 1/" from the first lever. Again, push downward on your lever, to pop the bead away from its seat in the rim. If you can't do this, move your lever a half-inch closer to the first lever. Now continue to work the bead away from the rim all around the wheel, until you have one complete side of the tire off the rim. Then, using your spoon from the opposite side of the wheel, work the second bead off the rim. (You are now working the bead off the rim-side away from you, as of course both beads must come off the same side to free the tire.) Taking one side of the tire off at a time is much easier than trying to force both beads off at once.

Note: when you begin working with the first tire lever, be sure to start at a point on the wheel opposite to or at least away from the valve stem. Also, new tires are a bear to remove the first time, so expect difficulty.

f) Take the tube out of the tire and check the outside and inside of the tire for embedded glass, pebbles, thorns, etcetera. When you are sure that it is clear, move on to the tube. I have had only two holes in my life which leaked so little that I was forced to hold them under water to look for air bubbles. All the other times I merely pumped up the tube and listened for escaping air. (Once. I heard air coming out of the center of the valve. If you look at a tube valve carefully you will see that the inside is threaded. If this core is not screwed into place tightly it will result in a leak. The proper tool to tighten a valve core is the valve cover tool. a tiny slotted metal cap which you should buy to replace the worthless black plastic caps present on all the tubes sold. If you have a very slow leak. check that your valve core is tight before you remove the wheel from the frame.)

g) Once the hole is located you can rough up the area with the patch kit scraper. Be sure to do a good job of it, short of putting additional holes in the tube, and be sure to roughen an area a bit larger than the size of the patch.

h) Apply the glue, again a bit more than necessary to cover the patch area. Most kits suggest waiting until the glue is dry to apply the patch. So, wait. Hurry this step and there's a good chance you'll be taking the wheel back off the bike a few miles down the road. Be careful not to touch the patch side which goes on the tube, and once in place, press the edges of the patch with a tire spoon.

i) If you have done all things properly thus far, you can reassemble the wheel immediately and ride on. But, before you do, check that the 'tape' is in place. This is the usually black rubber or cloth wrapping which sits on the rim covering the spoke ends. If you remove the tape you can see spoke nipple ends; spokes of the wrong length would protrude through the tape and into the tube. Spokes of correct length, when adjusted for alignment, or, just by the normal tension produced when riding, sometimes twist up past the nipple top. The tape protects the tube from the resultant punctures. Replacement tapes, if you break one, are available at bike shops or from catalogues. I have used a piece of scotch tape and even a staple in the past for repair, and gauze as replacement one time on tour.

J) Pump up the tube slightly, so that it can easily be placed inside the tire, without fear of wrinkles in the rubber. Once the tube is replaced, push the valve stem through the hole in the rim. making sure that it is completely pushed through, and that it *remains* perfectly perpendicular to the rim at all times. Riders who fail to do this, or who ride with low air pressure in their tires (which causes the tube to shift and the valve stem to angle out of the hole), cause wearing of the stem along its side and base. Once a hole occurs in the valve stem the entire tube is shot, for stems cannot hold a patch.

With the stem in place, begin putting *one* side of the tire back on the rim. (At this point, when working with PR tubes, I release the air inside. It makes replacement easier.) When taking the tire off, you begin at a point opposite the stem; when replacing a tire you begin at the valve stem. You should be able to put one side of the tire back on the rim by hand alone, without spoons, though a new tire or inexperience may require their use. Once one side is fully in place, and again starting at the valve, tuck the other bead into its home in the rim.

You will end up with six inches or so of tire which seems to be far too short to stretch into place. But remember that the tire was on the same rim before, and that the name for this type of tire - clincher - is given for its ability to 'clinch' itself to the wheel. Use your spoon in the opposite manner to replace the tire, and use it with beveled-end down. If both beads are properly seated, and the stem is still perpendicular, inflate the tire to its desired pressure. Do this before you put the wheel back on the bike, for it will mean less to mess with if you have goofed with the patch. But don't worry. A chimp can master a patch kit.

k) If the tire remains hard for a minute, slap it back on your bike and pedal off. But, *do not forget to reset your brakes.*

2. Wheel alignment - 'truing' your wheels is an adjustment most successfully done with a stand made especially for this purpose. I must admit to not owning one, and never having owned one. In fact, I took my first cross-country ride without even knowing a wheel could come

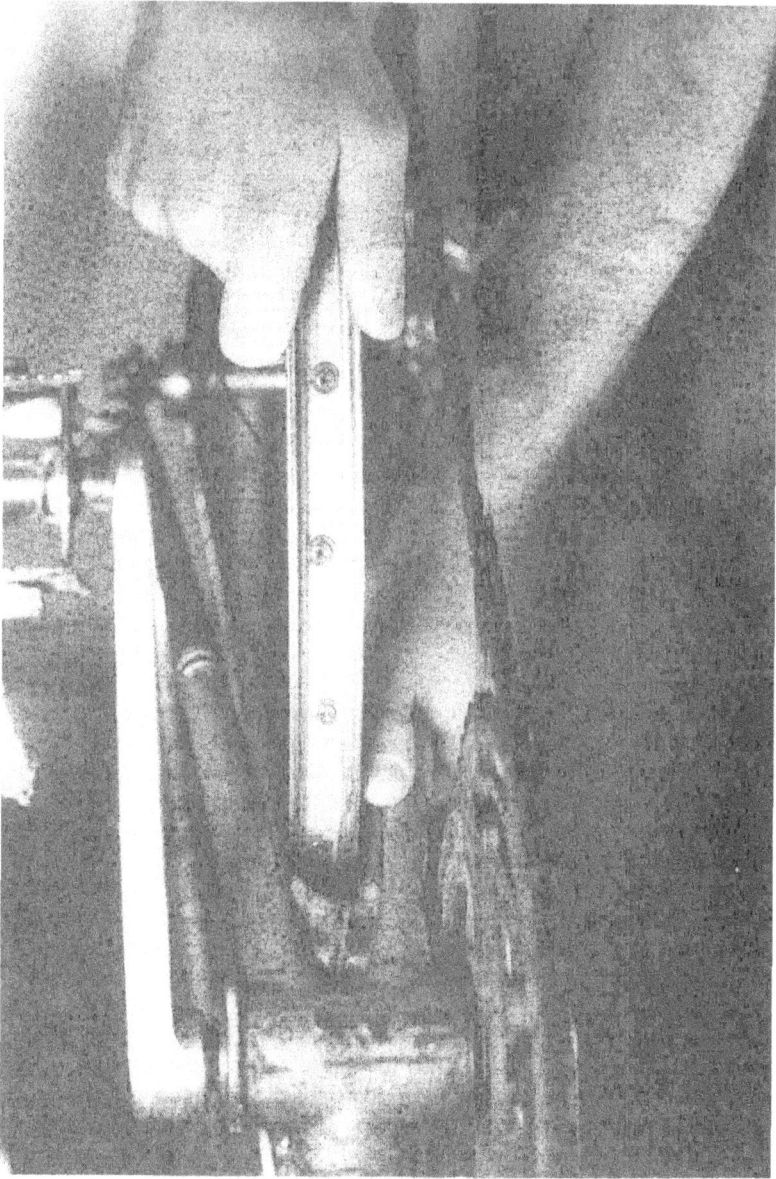

out of true. When I first had to align a badly battered wheel it was on the road, and of course without a truing stand within a hundred miles. And all the times since then when I've had to align my wheels it has been while on the road, on tour. So, I'll teach you my method, the one which will get you back home if you break down.

Wheels can be out of true in two ways; they can sway from side to side, and they can have high and low spots - which is referred to as being out of 'round'. Look closely at your wheel. Notice that the spokes reach out to the rim from both sides of the hub. Focus upon one spoke and think what tightening (shortening the length of) that single spoke will do. It should be obvious to you, if you are really thinking, that the rim will be pulled in two directions at the same time when the spoke is tightened, or moved *back* in two directions if loosened. Tighten the spoke and the rim will be 1) pulled closer to the hub, and 2) pulled in the direction of the side of the hub to which the other end of the spoke is attached. Loosen the spoke and the opposite movement will occur. Tighten a spoke which comes from the other side of the hub and the rim will move in *that* direction. As you can see, the spokes must be equal in tension to produce a 'straight' or 'true' wheel.

You may wonder why spokes ever come out of alignment. Ponder for a moment what the job of the unappreciated spoke is - and the enormous tension it is placed under. They are the most slender, delicate parts of your machine yet they are the major instrument of support for your body, all your gear, and the rest of the bike. Not only must they hold you up, and fly around and around at tremendous speeds, but they must balance you when you are wheeling around a tight curve at a 45 degree angle to the ground. Ever wonder why you don't fall over when you're doing that? Try keeping your feet pressed together; have a friend tilt you at a 45 degree angle, and see if you are still standing a second after he lets go. The reason a bike doesn't fall is the revolving wheels - the gyroscopic action applied when riding.

Now that you appreciate the spokes a bit more, let's get on to adjusting them. If you study a new wheel closely, running your hand along the spokes, you'll notice that they all appear to have the same amount of tension. Of course, that seems logical when you think of the need for the wheel to be held just as tightly by the spokes coming from one side of the hub as from the other, so that the wheel will be straight. If you were to break one spoke, or loosen one greatly, the wheel would be pulled harder to that side of the hub which still has all its spokes at proper tension. It's like a tug-of-war, with two sides pulling at a rope. When one side weakens, the rope (or rim) is pulled to the stronger side.

Normal riding over city streets will, in time, knock any spoked wheel out of true. How much time? Well, this depends upon your weight, road conditions, kind of spoke and hub, amount of 'dishing' (the degree to which the spokes on the right side of the rear wheel are 'flattened' to allow for the cluster space on the axle), and several other factors. When I'm on tour and carrying heavy loads I check my wheel alignment at least once a week. At home, I'm ashamed to say that usually I feel the sway of a misaligned wheel before I remember to check it. (Sort of like motorists neglecting the water level in the battery, until the winter morning when the engine won't turn over.) If I failed to correct the wobble I would in time snap a spoke, so let's deal with the small wobbles first.

I am yet to align a wheel by adjusting just one spoke. Generally, five or so must be worked with - and sometimes more. My method of truing is the following:

a. Take your tire, tube and tape off the wheel. (This allows for a more accurate truing, and exposes the screw head of the spoke nipple for adjustment with a screwdriver. It also allows you to see if too much spoke extends through the nipple head - a real danger to your tube.)

b. Place the wheel back on the bike. (Your bike is of course on its back.)

c. Spin the wheel with your hand, noting the wobble side-to-side. d. To determine the extend of the wobble, place your thumb next to the wheel rim (with the palm of your hand resting on the chainstay bar) so that your thumbnail lightly touches the rim at every point except for the wobble. At that point, the rim will reach out and smack your thumbnail - your job is to pull that wobble back into line with the rest of the rim.

e. Check the tension of the spokes in the area of the wobble. Chances are they'll be a bit more loose than the rest of the spokes in the wheel. Usually I am successful in tightening the spoke most at the center of the wobble, and less tightening for the other spokes as we move farther from the worst wobble point.

f. But how do you tighten a spoke? And what if two spokes appear to sit right smack in the middle of the problem area? Easy - just recall that spokes reach out to the rim from both sides of the hub. Naturally, tightening a spoke coming from the right side pulls the rim toward the right; from the left hub side, to the left. Say your wobble is to the right. You'll be tightening the spokes in that area of the rim which some from the left side of your hub. (I prefer to use a small screwdriver in the nipple slot head - and I always start off with a slight adjustment, about a half-turn for the spoke at wobble center, $1/4$ turn for spokes on either side, 1/8 turn for the next two spokes. You can also tighten spokes with a 'spoke nipple wrench', but the flat sides on these nipples tend to round-off quickly. Therefore, I only use the spoke wrench when I am adjusting spokes with the tire still on the rim something I only do in an emergency.)

g. On occasion you might have to loosen some spokes and tighten some others in the wobble area to produce a true wheel, especially if you have trued your wheel several times before. In loosening spokes follow the same pattern as above, more toward wobble center, less thereafter.

h. When your thumbnail-guide tells you all is well, you have two final things to do. First, check your spokes for approximately the same tension on all. You won't be perfect on this, but at least be close, or you'll be aligning your wheel again real soon. Secondly, step to the side of your bike, spin the wheel and check for its 'round'. If you have one high spot tighten the spokes slightly in this area - to pull the rim toward the hub a bit. But be sure to watch that you don't lose your side-to-side true as you do this.

i. I would like to add, as a postscript to wheel alignment, that this has got to be the most exasperating repair work on a bike. Take it easy, and keep your cool. Losing your temper will not force those spokes into place.

Bikers use the terms 'wobble' and 'blip' to denote different problems. 'Wobble' is corrected by spoke adjustment, as you have just learned. But 'blip' refers to a bulge in the rim, a condition which no amount of spoke alignment will eradicate. This problem usually results from riding with tires woefully underinflated, or from riding into huge potholes, sewer drains, trying to jump curbs, and so on. Luckily, I've never had a bad blip on my wheels (though I've dealt with more than my rightful share of broken spokes and wheel wobbles). However, on a rough ride through downtown St. Louis, my cycling companion once produced a real beauty on his rear wheel. Due to its size he was unable to keep his rear brakes applied when he needed to, for the brake pads touch on the very part of the rim where blips appear. We stopped at a service station to borrow a pair of vise-grips, and cut two thin shims of wood from an old paint can stir-stick. These pieces we placed next to the rim, inside the vise-grip jaws, then squeezed very carefully. This did the trick for us, but if you someday have a blip which remains on one side of the rim after the other side has been restored, or if a blip has appeared on only one side to begin with, place the wood shim on the flat side, and have a go at the fat blip with the metal jaw of the vise grip. *But,* squeeze gently, and watch both sides of the rim so that you do not push it past its proper profile.

3. Broken spokes - spokes need to be replaced when 1) they snap when you are riding, and 2) when the nipple heads are frozen in place on the spoke threads, refusing adjustment. In this second instance you'll just have to use the diagonal clipper portion of your needle-nose pliers to snap the spoke, and buy a new one.

You already know how to align your wheel, so don't let spoke replacement scare you. That is, unless you are in the middle of Hungary when you hear that terrible 'snap' in your rear wheel, see that you've lost a spoke on the freewheel side, and then recall that you don't have a freewheel puller in your tool bag. (This happened to Wayne and me in '74.) But we'll fix you up so you'll never be in that position.

Look closely at your hub and you will see that the spokes enter into spoke holes in an alternating pattern - every other spoke head will be visible when you view your hub from one side. Let's imagine you have neglected your wobbly rear wheel for so long that a spoke snaps on your way home from work. We'll go in steps through the repair process.

a. Get your cursing over as soon as possible - *before* you start the repair.

b. Stop riding your bike and fix it, for riding with one broken spoke soon causes a second break, and so on.

c. Remove your panniers, take out your tools and one of the extra spokes you carry at all times taped behind your seat tube - then flip your bike on its back.

d. Take off your rear wheel, remove the tire, tube, and rim tape. Remove the freewheel (see above). Then replace the wheel on the frame.

e. Remove the broken spoke. This is very easy, for spokes break at the bevel, and can then be taken out by pulling from the nipple end.

f. Take the nipple from the new spoke. Look at the rear hub, and concentrate on the next closest spokes to the one that broke. If you see two spoke heads next to the empty hole in the hub you know that your new spoke must enter from the other side, to follow the alternating pattern around the entire hub. Guide the spoke into the hole. (Don't be afraid to bend the spoke a bit.) Once it is completely through, look at the next closest spoke which enters the hub in the same direction as your replacement spoke. This will be your guide on lacing your replacement - how many spokes you must cross, and which to go over or under with the new spoke. (You'll have to bend the spoke even more here - be sure to bend it along its entire length, thereby not putting a crimp in it.)

g. Put the nipple into the rim, and thread the new spoke into it. Tighten the spoke until it is approximately the same tension as the rest, then align the wheel.

h. Check to see that the new spoke shaft does not protrude past the nipple. If it does, use the metal file of your Swiss Army Knife (a constant companion in your tool bag) to file it down.

i. Replace rim tape, tube, tire; inflate, and ride on.

j. Realize that if you looked after your alignment once in a while you wouldn't have broken the spoke to begin with.

4. Wheel bearing maintenance - bearing maintenance on a bike -cleaning and lubricating old bearings, or replacing them if necessary -is a procedure which I go through twice a year (more often if my touring takes me along many dirt roads). The entire operation, including the bearings in the crankset, takes about two hours. And for this investment of time I have a machine which rolls beautifully and pedals easily. As with all mechanical directions the operation seems impossibly difficult at first. But stay with it, master the only difficult part of cone adjustment, and you'll be one step further toward independence on the road. We'll begin with front wheel bearings.

a. As you can see in the diagram, a front wheel hub consists of a hub shell, two sets of bearings, two dust caps, an axle, two cones, two keyed lockwashers, and two lock nuts. (Add to this your quick-release mechanism, or large axle nuts and washers which hold the wheel on the frame).

b. Remove the front wheel from the bike, and take off the frame-mounting axle nuts and washers, or the quick-release. (The latter may be removed by holding the handle side fast, while unscrewing the other 'bale-nut' end. Notice the two cone-shaped springs which are held in place on the axle by the handle and bale-nut - be sure to replace them later in the same direction as they were originally, with smaller end toward hub, larger toward fork blade.)

c. Holding the locknut on one side of the hub with a crescent wrench, use a second wrench to loosen the locknut on the opposite hub side. Unscrew the locknut completely, putting it somewhere so that you'll not kick it as you continue working. Next remove the keyed lockwasher. (The term 'keyed' is used to denote the small pointed

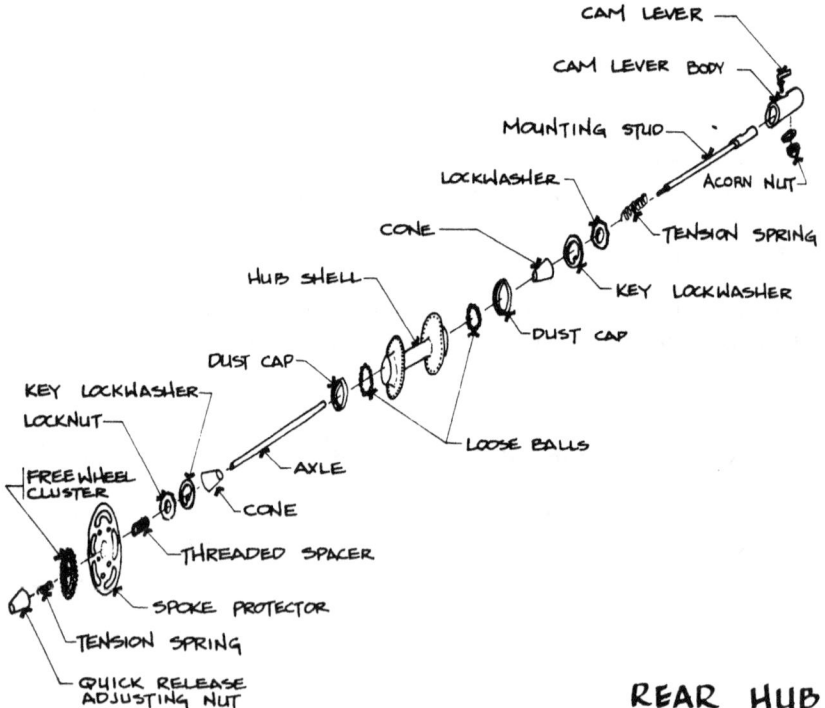

REAR HUB

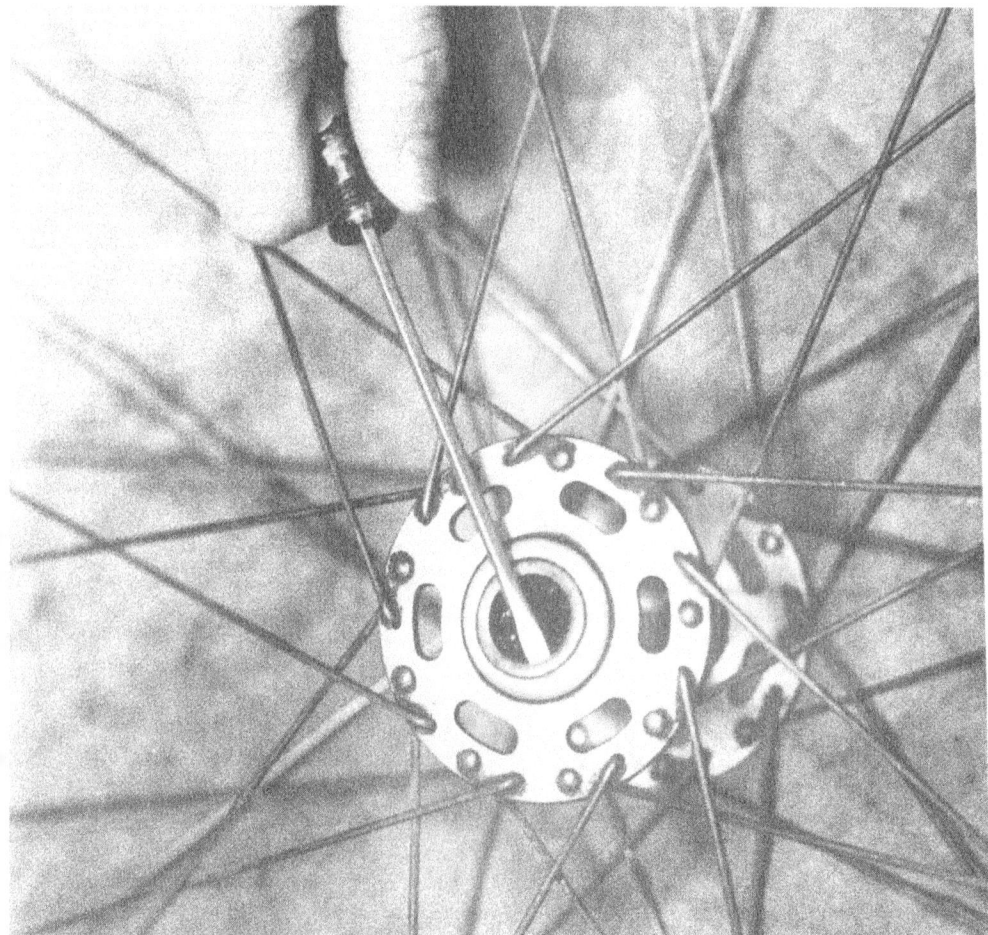

flange of metal on the inside of the washer - which fits into the groove on the axle.)

d. You are now to the cone, the place named for its tapering end which rests against the bearings. To adjust the amount of pressure placed on the bearings by this cone, the other end of the cone is squared for a 'cone wrench' - a very thin wrench which should be used for no other mechanical purpose that for which it was designed. (It will last you a life time if you treat it right-just like your bike.) Take hold of the squared-off end with the cone wrench and back it off the axle completely.

e. When this is done you have freed one side of the axle, and are free to pull the other axle side out of the hub. Do so, watching for small bearings which might fall out.

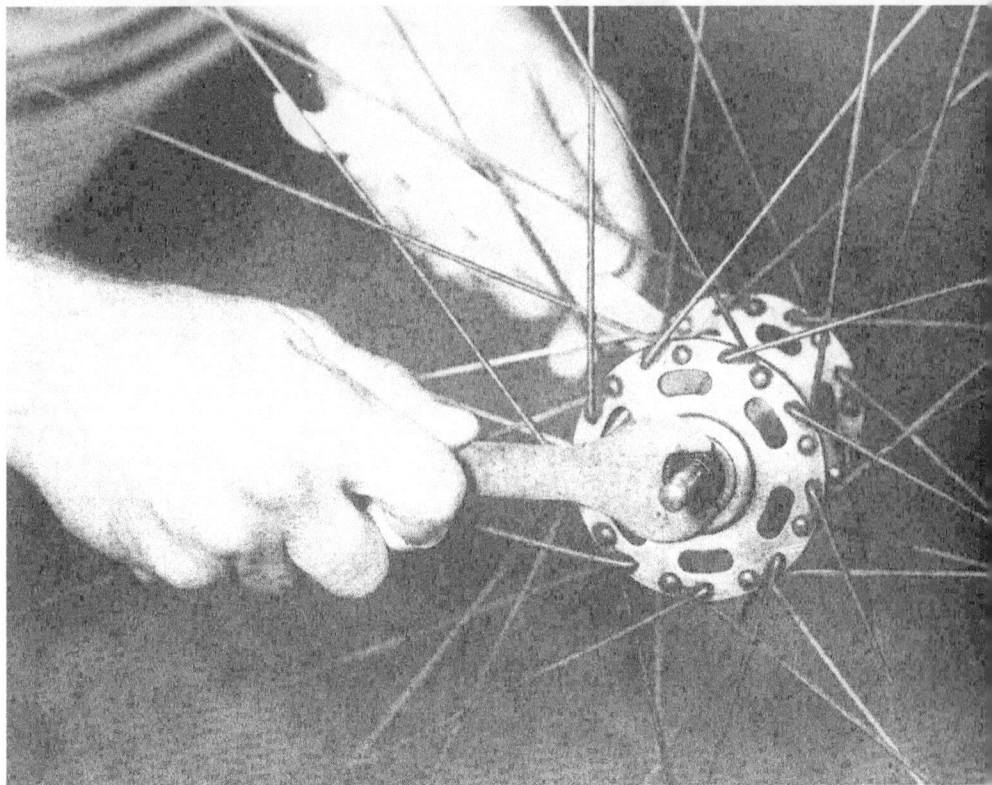

f. Now, take a small screwdriver and place the flat edge beneath the dust cap on the hub. This cap is designed to hold the bearings in place, and to fit so snugly into the hub as to keep out water and dirt. Therefore, it will be difficult to remove, and you may have to lift the cap in several places with the screwdriver before it comes out.

g. With the dust cap gone, look at your bearings. If you are pulling frequent maintenance there will be grease covering them still; this is a good sign that you've not waited so long that damage to your components might have occurred. Count the bearings, and notice, before you remove them, the small space present - bearings are not supposed to be wedged tightly into place. Now remove the bearings, cleaning and inspecting each individually for pitting or cracks. Bearings cost about 70 cents for a bag of twenty or more; a single hub costs from $20 on up. If you save a few cents by keeping cracked or pitted bearings you'll lose dollars in the end with a pitted hub. So replace them when they need it. (Be sure to buy a bag of each size bearing you might need before you break down your wheel. Otherwise you'll be walking to the bike shop.) Bearing sizes fall generally into the following categories:

3/16" -front hubs

1/4" - rear hubs, bottom brackets
1/8" - freewheel
5/32" - pedals, headsets

h. Once both dust caps and all bearings are removed and cleaned, take out the grease remaining in the hub, and wipe it clean with a cloth. Do the same to the underside of each dust cap. You are now ready to rebuild your wheel.

i. Apply a bead of fresh grease to the bearing cup of one side of your hub. Replace the bearings; then cover them with a second liberal bead of grease. Replace the dust cover by tapping it lightly with a small tack hammer, though any tool with a bit of weight and a flat side will do -when on the road I use the 6" crescent wrench.

j. Take the axle (which still has the cone, lockwasher and locknut on one side) and insert it into the hub side in which you have just replaced the bearings. Be sure to have cleaned and checked the cones -for they too are far less expensive to replace than an entire hub. Now you can turn your wheel over and replace the bearings in the other side, for the dust cap and cone will keep the bearings from falling out.

k. Once the bearings are in place around the axle on this second side, replace the dust cap, thread the cone finger-tight against the bearings, slide on the lockwasher, and screw on the locknut. Your hub is now rebuilt, but not ready to be ridden, for the cones have not been adjusted to the proper pressure against the bearings. Too loose, and the wheels will roll from side to side, ruining your bearings and cup and cone in time. Too tight, and the wheel will not roll properly.

l. Use the cone wrench to back off the cones a quarter turn or less if, when you turn the axle, it does not revolve easily in the hub. (The wheel is still off the bike.) What usually happens is that a person will back off the cones too far, creating side-play. This is when the axle moves back and forth in the hub. Even a slight amount of movement will be greatly accentuated when the wheel is replaced on the frame, so try to remove the side-play while still retaining free rolling movement of the axle. Just when you think you've got the best of both worlds, tighten the locknuts on both sides. (Hold one side fast with a crescent wrench or in a vise while tightening the other side.) The first time you do this you will notice that you have tightened the cone against the bearings somewhat by snugging the locknuts - and you'll have to readjust the cone once more. But don't get angry. Merely hold the locknut on one side of the axle fast with your crescent wrench, while backing off the same side cone ever so slightly with your cone wrench. This is usually sufficient for me to align it properly; but if not perfect just back off the locknut a quarter-turn and try again. Expect it to be difficult at first, and *much* easier the second time.

m. Once side-play is absent, and the axle moves freely, replace the quick-release or axle washers and nuts, and restore the wheel to the frame. Once it is secured, spin the wheel and check again for rolling ease and for side-play. If it is *not* correct do not sell your bicycle. Go upstairs or into the house, yell at your spouse or kick the dog, and then return to your bike and adjust your cones once more. But don't give up, and above all do not ride it if you still have side-play.

5. Freewheel removal - the only difference in bearing maintenance for the front and rear wheels is the need to remove the freewheel. Do so by following these steps:

a. When you purchase your bike, ask the shop owner which type of freewheel you have - Sun Tour, Shimano, Regina, etcetera. Buy the proper freewheel removal tool (less expensive in bike catalogues - Sun Tour $4, Shimano $4.80, Regina $5.90), for it will ride with you always in your tool bag.

b. Once you have the proper tool, and when you must remove the freewheel to replace a broken spoke on the cluster side, or wish to pull maintenance on your rear wheel bearings, remove the wheel from

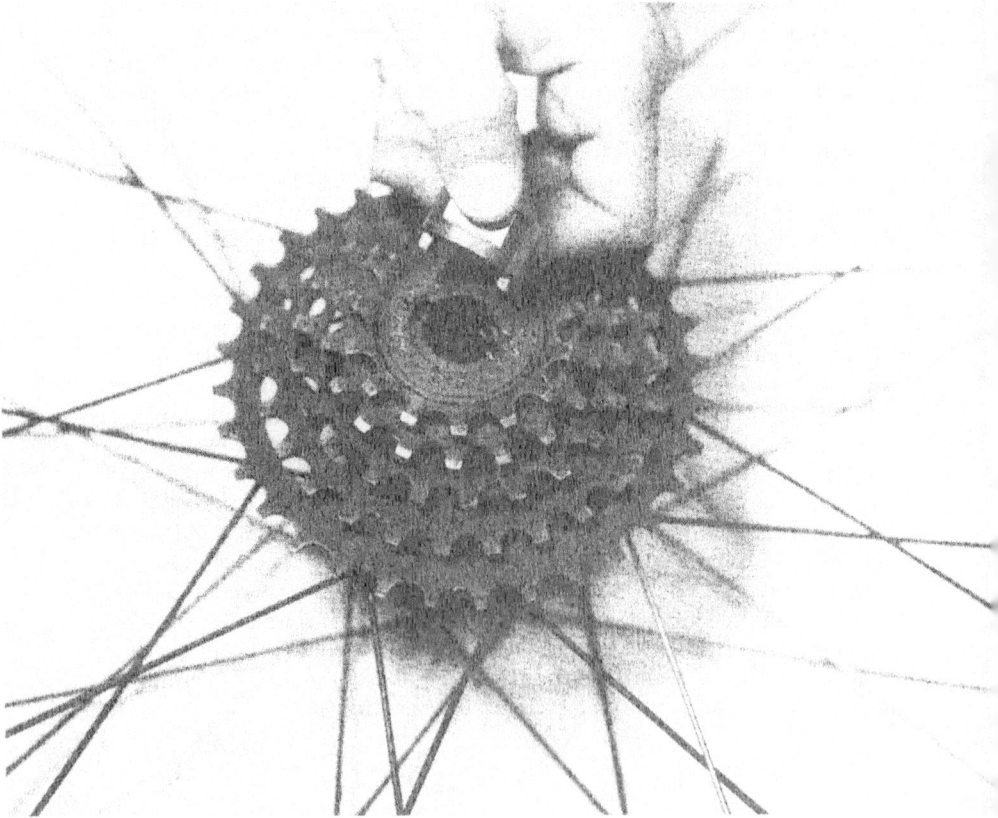

your bike and take off the axle nuts and washers (or quick-release mechanism). Look inside your freewheel. You will see either splines or two notches. Slip the freewheel tool onto the axle and see if it will engage the splines or notches on the tool securely. If not, and if you have the proper tool, the problem is the presence of a 'threaded spacer' blocking your tool's descent into the freewheel. Screw off this spacer from the axle.

c. If you have access to a vise you are well off, for this is the easiet method I know of. Take the freewheel tool and clamp it tightly in the vise. (You will see one flattened side for this purpose.) Next, set your wheel on the tool, making sure the splines or notches engage properly. When engaged, take hold of the wheel at the 3 and 9 o'clock positions from where you stand, and turn the wheel counter-clockwise. This will be difficult, especially if you are a strong rider. Once the freewheel gives way you can continue the counter-clockwise movement until you feel the wheel separate from the freewheel, or lift the wheel from the vise and finish unscrewing the freewheel by hand.

What do you do if no vise is around? If home, or in the vicinity of a service station, you can use what I purchased some time ago and have removed dozens of freewheels with - a 15" crescent wrench. (Once, under duress, I used a large pipe wrench, but I don't suggest it.) Place the removal tool in the crescent's jaws as tightly as possible. Stand over your wheel, the freewheel on the right, your left hand at the top of your rim. Engage the removal tool and freewheel securely, and position the wheel so that the wrench handle angles up toward you, not away from you. Take hold of the wrench and push down on it, being careful not to allow the removal tool to slip out of the free-wheel. With the application of a good deal of pressure the freewheel will 'break', and then you can easily thread it off the wheel.

Finally, what do you do if you aren't near a vise or a large crescent or pipe wrench when a spoke on the freewheel side snaps? For this terrible situation I carry a small channel-locks wrench, only 5W long overall. This I use in the same manner as the 15" crescent, though with some modification. First, in order to hold the freewheel tool securely in the jaws of the channel-locks I use a shock cord wrapped around the handles of the wrench. Next I fold a piece of cloth (bandana, sock, T-shirt), over the handle, to save my palm once I begin applying the great force necessary to remove the freewheel with such a small tool. And then I follow the steps described above with the crescent.

d. When the freewheel is off, you may find a metal or clear plastic 'spoke protector' ready to fall off as well. (This is held in place only by the freewheel.) The purpose of this disc is implied by the name: it guards the spokes from the chain if you greatly overshift into your largest sprocket in the rear. Personally, I do not like the looks of the disc, I begrudge the extra weight, and I keep my rear derailleur aligned so as not to worry about such extreme overshifting. I remove my spoke protector disc completely, and do not replace it when rebuilding the wheel.

e. You are now free to pull maintenance on your rear wheel bearings just as you did with the front hub.

Cotterless Crank

You may recall the discussion of cranks in the first chapter, when I pleaded with you to purchase a crank without a cotter pin and explained why. I am assuming that you took my advice, or purchased a cotterless replacement for your old bike, and therefore will discuss only the maintenance of the *cotterless* crank.

Note in the diagram the various parts of the crank assembly. In our discussion the 'right-hand' side will refer to the chainring side, the 'left-hand' side to the crankarm without a chainring. Remove, service, and replace your cotterless crank in the following manner.

a. Read the brand name of your crank assembly, or better yet ask your bike shop dealer when you buy your bike. Then, in the bike shop or through the bike catalogues, purchase the appropriate crankarm removing tool (small enough for carrying in your tool bag, also good for home use - between $4 and $8), or a 'universal' crank tool set for approximately $20 (too heavy to carry on the road). The removing tools consist of a wrench to pull the crankarm fixing bolt, and the puller assembly itself. When you have the proper tool you may begin servicing your crank.

b. Remove your crankarm dust caps. This can be done with a screwdriver blake on some, and a small alien wrench with others.

c. Remove the crankarm fixing bolts and washers. Most removal tools have one side which slips around the fixing bolt head, with the other end beveled to accept a large crescent wrench. Two of the removal tools, the Sugino Mighty and the Stronglight, have a small breaker bar to take the place of a crescent wrench.

d. Carefully screw the crankarm puller into the crankarm, making sure that the threads meet perfectly. Use your wrench to snug this puller into place.

e. Now insert the extractor portion of the tool into the puller. At first it will move freely, then stop when it reaches the crank spindle (axle). Use your large crescent wrench to turn the extractor gently, and you will see (if you are working first with the right-hand side) the chainrings begin to slip off the spindle toward you. Lift the chain off the chainring and place it out of the way on the spindle housing.

CRANK ARM

MOUNTING BOLT

LOCKRING

ADJUSTING CUP

WASHER

BALL RETAINER

STATIONARY CUP

PEDAL SPINDLE

BALL RETAINER

CRANK ARM AND SPROCKET

WASHER

MOUNTING BOLT

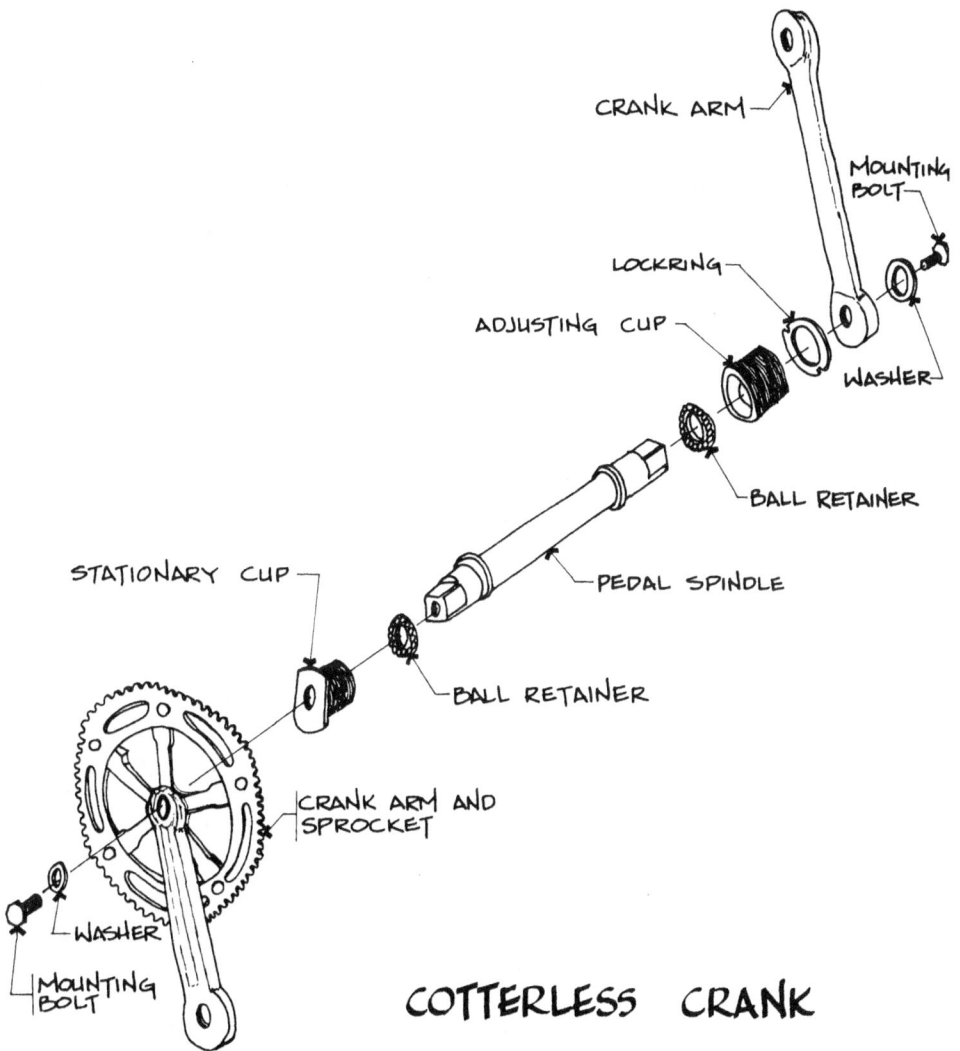

COTTERLESS CRANK

Remove the left-hand crankarm in the same way.

f. Look closely at both sides of your crank spindle. The right-hand side is held by a 'fixed' bearing cup which is squared-off to accept the large crescent wrench for removal. The left-hand side has an 'adjustable' cup which must be removed with either an adjustable cup tool ($8 - $12) or a punch and hammer. (In a bind on tour you can use the edge of a screwdriver as a punch, or the leather punch or fish hook dis-gorger on your Swiss Army Knife.) The fixed cup is merely threaded completely into the bottom bracket; the adjustable cup is what you will adjust so as once again to apply only the correct pressure against the bearings. The adjustable cup is held in place by a lockring.

g. Use the crescent wrench or a fixed cup tool (approximately $10, usually with a lockring tool on the other end) to remove the fixed cup, but only once you've put something beneath to catch the bearings should they fall out. (If they don't fall out they are probably held in a 'ball-retainer' or 'bearing-race'. This is a small circular metal holder which allows the bearings to revolve freely inside.) Once the fixed cup is removed take out the spindle. Notice it has one longer side. This side will be replaced later so as to point toward the chainring.

h. You must first remove the lockring before you can take off the adjustable cup. This is most easily accomplished with a lockring tool, which is properly notched to fit the edges of the lockring. On the road I use a screwdriver blade with something similar to a hammer - the palm of my hand, a piece of wood, a large rock. Back the lockring off the cup completely. Then, using your adjustable cup tool or punch and hammer, remove the adjustable cup from the bottom bracket. Clean, inspect, and replace if necessary all the ball bearings. Wipe all surfaces clean.

i. Apply a generous bead of grease on the inside of your fixed bearing cup, replace the bearings, and cover them with a second layer of grease. Now thread this cup back into the frame (right-hand, chainring side), snugging it with your crescent wrench. (To insure easy removal some months in the future, I always rub a bit of lubricant over the threads inside the bottom bracket before replacing the cups.)

j. Lubricate and replace the bearings in the adjustable cup in the same manner, but do not thread the cup into place yet.

k. Take the cleaned spindle, longer side toward the fixed cup, and, from the other side of the bike (left side) carefully guide it through the bracket and fixed cup. If you have applied a good amount of grease, if your aim with the spindle is accurate, and if you have been kind to motorists all week, you won't knock any of the bearings out of place.

l. While holding the spindle end in one hand, pick up the adjustable cup, engage the spindle in the cup hole, and thread it into the frame. Stop threading this cup when it engages the bearings, and check for side-play in the spindle. If it is present, thread the cup a bit further, but not so far as to prohibit the free turning of the spindle.

m. When the adjustment is correct, replace the lockring, then re-check for proper bearing adjustment.

n. Replace both crank arms by slipping them onto the spindle, and tightening the fixing bolts. These must be secured well, and should be checked for tightness once every 40 or 50 miles for the next 200 miles.

o. Re-engage your chain on the chainring, and replace your dust caps.

Pedals

I have never had difficulty with pedals, or known anyone who did. And, as a result of such good performance, pedals are often neglected. They, too, have bearings which should be serviced, and as you can see in the diagram are very similar to the mechanics of a wheel axle (except for having a pedal instead of a hub between the cones). Since the method of servicing is so similar to wheel bearing lubrication, I will be brief.

a. I service my pedals while they are still on the bike, though you can remove them with a very thin crescent or open end wrench - thin enough to fit between the pedal body and the crank arm. Special pedal wrenches (usually with a bottom bracket fixed cup remover on the tail end) are available for $7, but are too heavy for the road. Once you have a wrench which will fit, merely back out the pedal spindle from the crank arm. The left pedal spindle backs out clockwise; the right is removed counter-clockwise.

b. Remove the pedal dust cap. Some of these caps have serrated

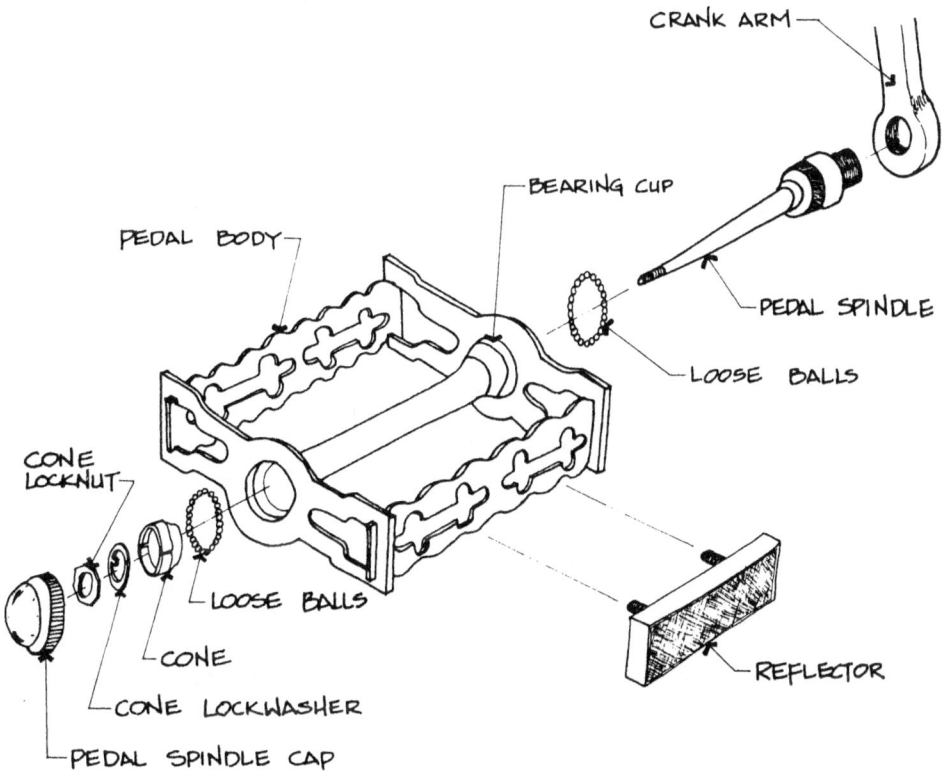

CRANK ARM

BEARING CUP

PEDAL BODY

PEDAL SPINDLE

LOOSE BALLS

CONE LOCKNUT

LOOSE BALLS

CONE

CONE LOCKWASHER

PEDAL SPINDLE CAP

REFLECTOR

PEDAL

edges to allow for easy gripping, but most have an hexagonal head which may be gripped with your crescent or small channel locks, or more easily with a pedal dust cap wrench ($2.25). This handy wrench only weighs an ounce, but is still too heavy for me to ride with, as other tools which I carry will do the job.

c. Remove the locknut and keyed washer, exposing the cone.

d. Due to the pedal housing you cannot get a wrench on the cone; the cone therefore has slots cut in its side (the side facing you) for your screwdriver. Using your small screwdriver blade, back out the cone.

e. Remove the cone, catching all bearings. Slip off the pedal, clean, inspect, and lubricate the bearings, bearing cups and cones.

f. Reassemble. Adjust cone for proper pressure against bearings in the same manner as described in wheel maintenance - free rotation of pedal but no side-play.

Brakes

After worrying about alignment of cones and proper spoke tension, brakes should be relatively simple. One reason is that all parts can be seen readily, and the operation of the brake is easy to understand after just a few minutes of study. You will see the cable leading from the hand brake to one side of the side-pull brake, or to the center of the center-pull. When the hand brake is squeezed, the cable is pulled away from the brake, causing the brake arm or arms to react to the cable tug. The reaction is, of course, a movement of the brake pads against the wheel rim, which slows the wheel's revolving speed and eventually stops the bike.

You should be able to see the two critical points with brakes. First, the cable must not be so loose as to prohibit a firm pressure against the rim by the brake pads when the brakes are applied, not so tight that the wheel rim is kept from revolving freely when the brakes are not set. Secondly, the brake pads must be in good shape and be positioned so that they strike the rim properly. Aside from an occasional drop of oil on the brake arms when they appear to be sticking (about twice a year), all of my maintenance work on brakes consists of adjusting or replacing the brake cable, and adjusting or replacing brake pads. So let me step you through these repairs.

1. Cable adjustment - almost all good multi-speed bikes today come equipped with an apparatus whereby a brake cable may be lengthened or shortened without the use of a tool, indeed, even while one is riding along. This is facilitated by an 'adjusting barrel' of some sort, and is in one of three positions - at the top of the brake arm for side-pull, directly above the center-pull by several inches, or just above the brake hoods on either model. This adjusting barrel or sleeve will

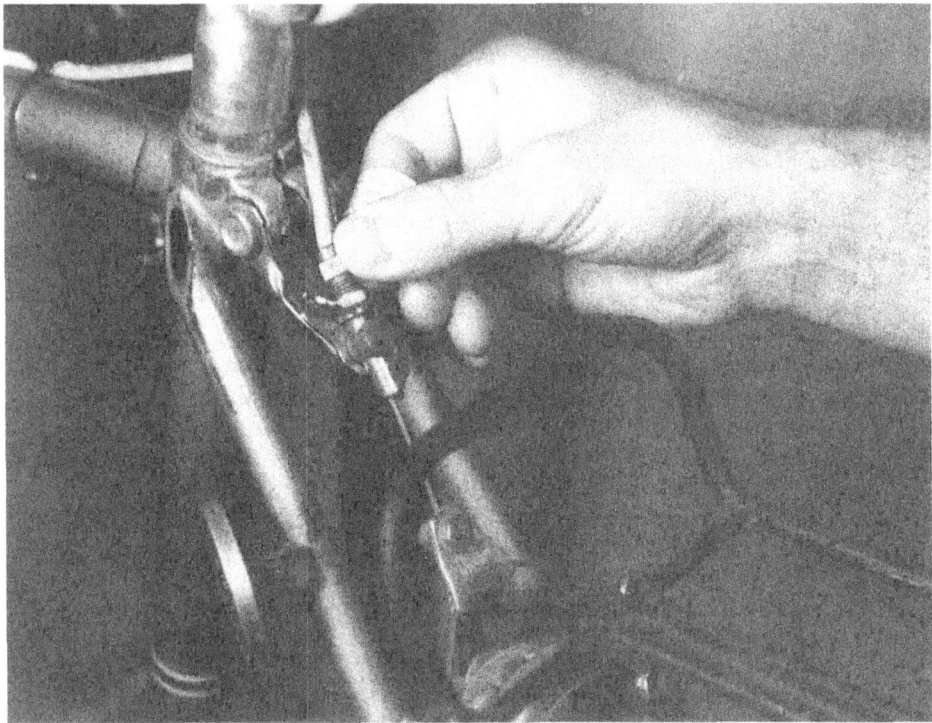

shorten a cable when it is turned counter-clockwise, therefore moving the brake pads closer to the rim. There is a locknut or lockring present beneath the barrel which must be loosened to allow the barrel to be moved, and re-tightened when the adjustment is made to hold the barrel in its new position.

Occasionally, the amount of cable adjustment necessary is beyond that allowed by the adjusting barrel. When this is so I first screw down the barrel completely, then apply a 'thirdhand' tool ($1.10). This tool fits around the acorn nuts on either brake pad (the nuts on the outside of the pad), holding the pads against the rim to allow much greater ease in changing the cable setting. When on the road I of course do not have this with me, so I ask a fellow cyclist to help, or merely do it myself in twice the time. When the tool or friend is in place, or when you are stumbling along by yourself, loosen the anchor bolt which holds the cable in place. (This bolt has a small hole in it, through which the cable runs.) Use your needle nose pliers to pull the cable tight, then tighten your anchor bolt once more. Center-pull brakes have a 'carrier' which holds the short transverse cable, and the anchor bolt is located here. Once the brake cable is held fast again by the anchor bolt, release the brake arms. I like the brake pads to rest no further from the rim than necessary to prevent constant rubbing. (This allows for very quick stopping in city riding.) If the brake pads are too close or too far from the rim, re-adjust the cable setting.

2. Cable replacement - some day you'll snap a brake cable, and will be happy that you always have one with you in your bike bag. I prefer to use my little 4" crescent for brake work, though a 6" will suffice. This tool, and the side-cutter portion of your needle nose pliers are all you'll need to replace a brake cable. (Cables run from 60 cents to $1.)

a. Stand in front of your bike and squeeze one of your brake levers. Look inside, and you'll see a screw head. This is what holds the brake lever on the handlebar. (If it becomes loose use a screwdriver to tighten it.) As you look at the screw head you'll notice your brake cable running in front of it. It is held in place by the barrel or ball end of the cable, which catches the hole or notch inside your brake lever. This hole is designed for either the barrel or ball end, so look to see which type you have by checking out your old cable. Many brake cables come with a barrel on one end, and a ball on the other, so that you will be sure to have the right kind with you at all times. (Bikecology now offers a "pear end" cable which they claim will work in place of both.)

b. Remove the old cable. Cut the end which you don't need off the new cable, and run a few drops of oil over the entire length. Reaching beneath your brake lever, guide the cut end through the barrel or ball slot in the brake lever, then into the plastic cable housing. This will be easier if you have cut the cable so as not to produce a frayed end.

c. When the cable comes out the other end of the housing, guide it through the adjustable sleeve and measure for the proper length by following the steps in brake cable and adjustment above. Secure it with the anchor bolt, and cut off excess cable.

Note - sometimes in winter riding, brakes and derailleurs will refuse to work, yet not appear faulty when they are inspected. The problem may well be a frozen cable due to cracked cable housing allowing moisture to enter and freeze up. I spend as little money on my bike as is mechanically wise, and therefore merely tape around small housing cracks. But if it is really battered after several years hard use I do replace it, being careful to cut it without smashing the interior steel casing. Work the diagonal blade of your needlenose in between the wound steel casing so that you are cutting only a single turn of metal. Cost of cable housing runs from 35 cents to $1 per foot.

3. Brake pads - the brake 'shoe' includes the metal housing and the pad. One development of late which greatly irritates me is the apparent preference of bike manufacturers to sell one-piece shoes. In other words, when a pad wears out the metal housing is tossed as well, unlike the two-piece kind which only requires a new pad. This Detroit throw-away mentality is a real motorist intrusion into the more sane world of cycling, and I lament it. So, if you demand two-piece shoes you'll not only save yourself considerable money over the next few decades, but help stop such a waste of machined metal.

Even with my year-round riding in city traffic I find that my brake pads last about ten to twelve months. Pads have a rubber block portion which appears squared off, and a smaller portion which reaches out to the rim. When your pad is wearing close to the 'block' portion: replace it; or earlier if it doesn't seem to be doing its job. Pads by themselves run from 50 cents to $2 apiece. (I use the 50 cent kind.)

In replacing your pads, you must watch out for several things. First, be sure to remount the metal brake shoe so that the *closed* end is toward the front of the bike. Why? Because the wheels revolve in a forward direction, and will otherwise shoot the pads right out of their metal holders when you squeeze the brakes. Secondly, make sure the pad hits the rim. Some folks say a squeaking brake can be corrected by very gently twisting the brake arm inward with a wrench so that the front of the pad touches the rim first. But I've never done it. All my brake squeaks have been ended by me cleaning my rims of grease and dirt. Most commercial cleaners will work on the rim, as will alcohol, turpentine, kerosene, and gasoline. Just don't get these substances on your tires. They eat rubber.

By the way, the pads will be real difficult to take out of the metal shoe. I hold on to the metal stud with my small channel locks or needlenose and place the pad against something immobile. Then, I push mightily against the open, metal end, and reverse the process to replace them.

Finally, sometimes I find my pads almost black with dirt. When they fail to clean up with alcohol I use the metal file on my Swiss Army Knife, and actually file off 1/16" or so of rubber. It works beautifully, and has kept me from shelling out 50 cents several times over the last decade. Don't laugh. It mounts up - half a buck here and there over the years in hiking can soon add up to what it costs a motorist to fill his tank *once*

Derailleurs

Maybe I wouldn't appreciate derailleurs the way I do if I hadn't peered into the workings of a transmission long ago at my auto school. Many of my friends are afraid of their changers, and thus can never be thankful for their beautiful simplicity, and amazing longevity. If you have purchased a moderately good derailleur on a moderately good machine (per my earlier suggestions), you'll have to do nothing beyond the simple cleaning, lubricating, and adjusting of your changer to obtain very good performance. And all this can be done without taking your derailleur apart.

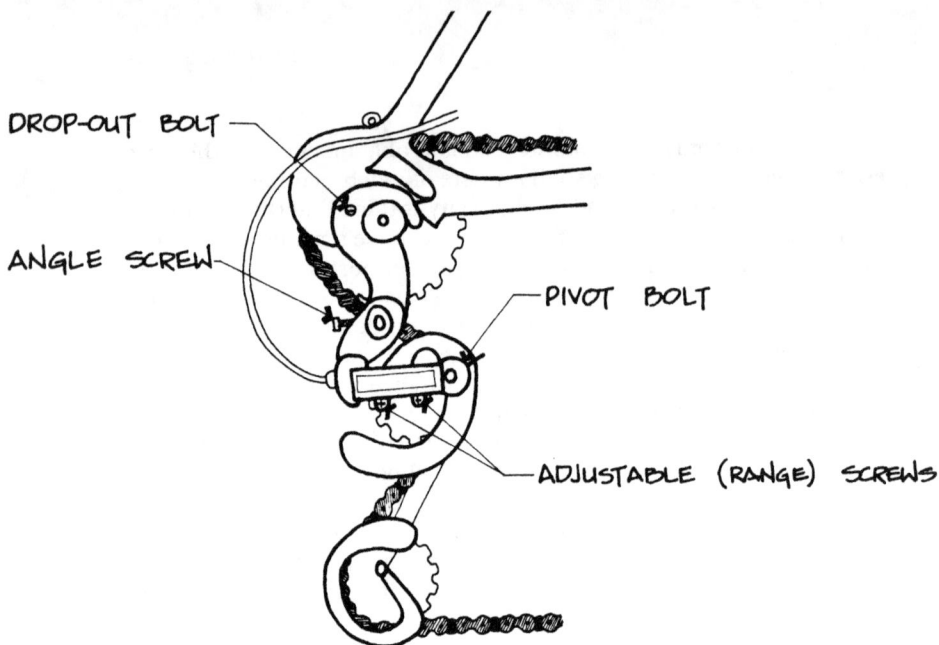

DROP-OUT BOLT

ANGLE SCREW

PIVOT BOLT

ADJUSTABLE (RANGE) SCREWS

REAR DERAILLEUR

I have suggested several times that anyone with an ability to read thoughtfully and think logically can, if they add a dash of patience, learn to maintain a bike. That goes for derailleurs as well. Look closely at the diagram and at your own bike as you read this. We'll start with the rear derailluer.

Basically, a gear cable runs from your shifters, along your down tube and chain stay, then through a familiar cable adjusting barrel, to a cable anchor bolt on your changer. When you pull back on your shifter lever you tighten the cable, which causes the derailleur to lift the chain from a smaller sprocket, and set it upon a larger one. Naturally, there are limits to how far in either direction you would wish your chain to go, and this limitation is established and maintained by 'high' and 'low' gear adjusting screws. The high gear screw keeps the chain from moving beyond the smallest sprocket and falling off the freewheel; the low gear screw keeps the chain from moving beyond the largest sprocket and attacking your spokes. The third screw present on some changers is an 'angle' screw. Chains, like cables, stretch in time, and thereby change the angle of the derailleur and thus its performance. This angle screw allows for taking up this tiny slack, by resetting the proper angle in relation to the freewheel. Below the derailleur housing are two pulleys, or rollers. Notice that the chain rolls over one, and under the second. The top pulley is the 'jockey' pulley - named this for its job of jockeying the chain into place over a sprocket. The bottom one is the 'tension' pulley, for it takes up the slack in the chain when the derailleur moves from a larger to a smaller sprocket. And the final thing you should notice - the points of lubrication. Simply apply two drops of oil every month to all springs and moving parts, then wipe off the excess. Now let's run through some very simple procedures which you'll need to follow when problems are encountered.

1. Your bike has fallen over in the mud on the derailleur side, or you haven't cleaned it for eight years now and it won't budge. *The solution:*

a) You are going to have to remove your changer from the bike, and clean it in a pan of some sort of solvent. (I use diesel fuel - a five gallon can of it was forgotten by the previous owners of our house. Kerosene and gasoline also work just fine.) Begin by loosening the cable anchor bolt, and removing the cable.

b) Most derailleurs I see today are affixed to the bike frame with a fork end bracket. One end of this bracket is bolted to the frame with a single bolt and locknut, the other end contains a large hole through which the pivot bolt is secured. (The pivot bolt allows the changer to dance back and forth as you change gears.) And the middle of the bracket is cut away to fit around the axle. You can remove your derailleur by backing out either the single drop-out bolt at the top of the fork end bracket, or the pivot bolt below. (I always remove the drop-out bolt, for unlike the pivot it has only a single locknut to worry about losing.)

c) On many derailleurs the chain will slip off the jockey and tension pulleys without having to disassemble the pulley cage. However, if yours traps the chain between the metal cage sides, remove the pulley spindles with your small crescent wrench. Then slip out the pulley, and allow your chain to hang free.

d) When the cable has been freed from the anchor bolt and adjusting barrel, the drop-out or pivot bolt removed, and the chain freed from the pulley cage, the derailleur is freed from the frame. Swish it about in your solvent, use an old tooth brush to clean the hard-to-reach areas, and pay particular attention to the internal springs if your changer has them.

e) If you have the type pulleys with ball bearings in them remove the cone bushings, clean, inspect, and lubricate the bearings. Reassemble by replacing bearings, threading the cone into the pulley by hand, and adjusting its pressure against the bearings as with all such operations above free rotation but no side-play. If your pulleys are like mine (without bearings), separate the metal bushing and side plates, clean and oil, and reassemble.

f) Wipe off all solvent from the derailleur, and allow to dry completely.

g) Oil all moving parts and springs, with two drops for the pivot bolt. Re-attach derailleur to bike frame with drop-out or pivot bolt, engage the chain and reassemble pulley cage if necessary. Thread the cable through the cable adjusting barrel and cable anchor bolt. This will be impossible if the cable end is badly frayed; a new cut may be necessary. With chain on smallest rear sprocket and larger front chain ring, pull the cable taut with your needlenose pliers, and tighten the cable anchor bolt. Do not pull the cable so taut as to move the derailleur. Also, the adjusting barrel should be screwed down all the way at this point; the barrel adjusts the cable by increasing the distance between the anchor bolt and barrel, and must be twisted counter-clockwise to do so. If the barrel is 'up' as far as it will go when the cable is first replaced, it will not be able to adjust the cable at all.

2. Your chain keeps slipping from larger to smaller sprockets. *The solution:*

a) The difficulty is usually located in your shifter assembly, not the derailleur. The shifters become loose after a while and need to be tightened. Remember the difficult job they have - they are under constant tension from the cable; they must be able to move easily in your hand when you shift gears, and yet must remain stationary once you have located them where you wish for the proper gear.

At the base of the shifter, where the attachment bolt is located, you will probably find a plastic wingnut of some kind. Some have a small wire bale, some only a slotted bolt head, large enough to be turned with a dime. The purpose of these special attachment bolts is to allow the rider to tighten the shifter arm if it moves by itself (in response to cable tension), or loosen it if so tight that shifting is difficult.

b) If the shifter is not causing the chain slippage, it is possible that the derailleur is at fault. Usually, in this case, it is a problem of a changer out of alignment, and the alignment of 'limiting' screws must be adjusted. (See below)

3. Your chain falls off the smallest sprocket, or jumps over the largest sprocket into the spokes, or won't quite move up enough to engage the largest sprocket, or down the freewheel to stay on the smallest. *The solution:*

a) Remember when I was explaining the simple operation of a derailleur, and I mentioned that it was of course necessary to limit the chain's side-to-side movement to the exact extent of the freewheel, to keep the chain from falling off in either direction? Well, if one or both of your 'chain-limiting' adjustment screws' are misaligned, you will have problems with your chain.

b) If the chain leaps over the largest sprocket, or cannot quite seat itself on this sprocket, your low gear chain-limiting screw must be adjusted. (Some derailleurs have a tiny 'L' for low gear, and 'H' for high gear stamped beneath the appropriate limiting screw.) Turning the screw clockwise with your small screwdriver will lessen the derailleur's movement, and therefore the chain's, in the direction of the largest sprocket. This will keep you from over-jumping the sprocket and hitting the spoke guard plate or spokes. Determine the degree of screw adjustment necessary by putting your bike on its back or in a stand, spinning your pedals and shifting. Turning the screw counter-clockwise will of course allow the chain greater freedom of movement toward the largest sprocket.

c) Adjustment of your derailleur for proper chain action on the smallest sprocket can be accomplished by turning the *high* gear limiting screw as necessary.

4. Your derailleur moves in response to you pulling back on the shifter (tightening the cable), but will not return to its original position when the shifter is moved forward again. *The solution:*

a) The problem could be, but probably isn't, a very dirty derailleur. The spring in the changer, if really loaded up with road grease, or frozen by rust, will hold the changer in one place no matter the shifter and cable movement. If this is so, clean and lubricate the entire derailleur, as described above.

b) Each time I've seen the problem of a derailleur which won't budge the solution has been to lubricate the cable. I mentioned earlier, in the discussion of brake cables, that a broken cable housing will allow water inside. This can freeze in winter, or cause rust any time of the year. So repair or replace cracked cable housing, and lubricate the dry cable with light oil to free it from sticking.

5. Your chain slips - not to another sprocket - but while on the same cog. *The solution:*

This has happened to me only once, and was not the fault of the derailleur. (I cover the problem here, however, because most people think at first that it is the derailleur.) The reason for my slippage was worn out sprocket teeth on the smallest cog in the rear. They didn't look all that rounded to me, but the tremendous torque applied to that little sprocket when pedalling in high gear over thousands of miles had worn it just enough. If you have this problem and determine that it isn't just a loose chain (by removing one of the links - see below in chain maintenance - or by pulling your rear axle as far back in the frame drop-outs as it will go), you may have to replace the sprocket or sprockets you normally ride in. How do you do this? It really isn't difficult, but it must be done with two tools too heavy to carry with you on the road. For this reason it is a good idea to begin very long tours with a new cluster. The following steps will guide you through freewheel sprocket replacement.

a) The disassembly may be done with or without the freewheel removed from the wheel. However, I think it is easier when apart (see above). You will need one sprocket tool if you have a vise, two sprocket tools if you do not. (These tools are merely a piece of chain riveted to the end of a steel rod - $7 per pair.)

b) Assuming you are using two sprocket tools, place the chain of one tool around the fourth sprocket down (second to largest), wrapping the chain in a clockwise direction. In the opposite direction wrap the chain of the second tool around the first (smallest) cog. I place these tools so that the handles are only a few inches apart. This allows greater control, for the handles must be pushed toward one another to unscrew the top sprocket. A strong rider's freewheel will require a great deal of strength to disassemble, for the first two sprockets are actually tightened on the freewheel body during pedalling. (When you are using two sprocket tools be careful not to apply uneven pressure against the handles - this will cause the entire freewheel to tilt and your tools will slip off. I've never damaged the tools or cogs when this happened, but I have run my knuckles into the sprocket teeth.) On most freewheels the first two sprockets screw off the freewheel body or 'core' in a counter-clockwise direction, and the three remaining cogs

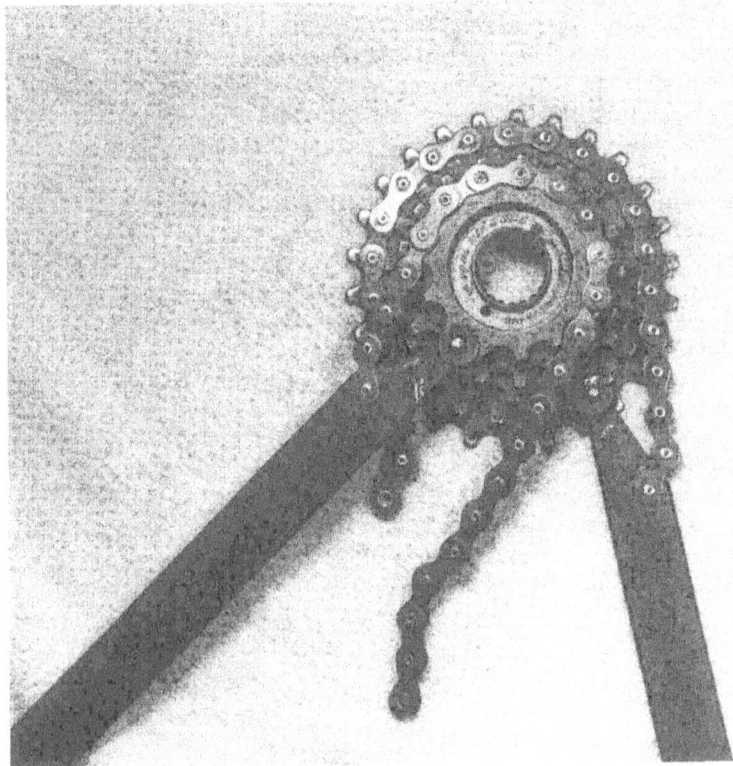

lift off. These last three have small lugs which fit notches in the core, and usually have spacer rings between them. Don't get the sequence mixed up when you take things apart - and with a freewheel you must also replace the sprockets with the same side up as you found them.

c) If you have a vise you can take your freewheel apart in two ways. First, grip the largest sprocket in the vise jaws, wrap the sprocket tool chain around the first cog in a counter-clockwise direction, and apply force to the handle. Then proceed with the remaining sprockets as described above.

Note: the second method (the use of a vise) requires a 'freewheel-axle vise tool' ($12). This tool holds the freewheel in a horizontal position for very easy disassembly.

d) To reassemble the freewheel, merely slip the first three sprockets and their spacers onto the body, and screw and tighten the top two in place. Reverse the direction of the sprocket tools to tighten the last two cogs.

Whereas some of my friends break down their freewheel bodies completely to clean and lubricate, I have never found this necessary, or worth my time to do so. The operation requires a pin spanner wrench and tweezers, and a great deal of patience to deal with the pawls and springs and tiny bearings inside. My 'road lubrication method' works well for me, and after many years, if the core goes bad, I can replace it for about $6. (Entire freewheels run from about $8.50 to $25.)

I clean my freewheel core by taking it off the wheel and laying it upside down (smallest sprocket to the ground) on newspaper. Then I flush the core with Liquid Wrench (4 oz. can - 69 cents). This is done by shooting the liquid between the dust ring and main body of the core - just inside the sprocket on the back side. Give the Liquid Wrench a few minutes to work through the bearings. Pick up the freewheel and move it to a dry piece of paper, then flush it a second time. (If the ball bearings inside the core were dirty the first newspaper will be dark with grease.) A third flushing may be necessary. Then allow the bearings to dry for a few minutes, and apply a fine, light bicycle oil.

Front derailleur

At first glance you will see that your front derailleur is more simple than the rear, but it is nevertheless woefully mistreated by insensitive riders. The damage occurs when a rider fails to move the 'cage' (chain guide) away from constant contact with the passing chain. I have actually seen cages with almost all of the inside metal arm eaten through. To keep yourself from ever ruining your derailleur cage and chain, look over the following problems and their solutions *before* a problem becomes too great.

1. You hear noise while pedalling, the sound of metal upon metal. *The solution:*

a) Don't 'learn to live with it'. One of the beauties of a bike is its silence. Besides, you'll soon be buying a new front derailleur and chain if you don't fix it.

b) Put your bike on a stand which elevates the rear wheel from the ground, or flip it on its back if you're on tour, or have a friend lift the back of the bike for you. Spin the pedals, and look to see when the chain hits the cage. It will probably do so at two times - when you are in your large chain ring and smallest rear sprocket, and again in your small chain ring and largest cog in the rear. (More often than not, the most severe damage is done to the inside arm of the cage.)

c) Once you determine where your chain is rubbing, look to see if the cage is perfectly parallel with the chain ring. If not, loosen the clamp bolt and turn the derailleur until it is so, being careful not to shift its position up or down on the seat tube. This *could* end your trouble. If it does not, or if the cage is parallel to the chain ring to begin with. locate the high and low gear adjusting screws.

d) If the rubbing takes place while you are on your large chain ring, adjust the high gear screw; only an eighth of a turn does wonders in derailleur work, so be careful not to overdo it. Turning the screw counter-clockwise will allow the cage to move out farther from the derailleur body. Adjust the screw until the chain moves freely during pedalling. However, you may have caused another common problem -the chain falling off the large front sprocket when shifting up from the smaller chain ring. Test for this problem by shifting a few times, and if the chain does fall off try the high gear adjusting screw again. If there appears no way to keep the chain from falling off *and* end the chain-cage contact, you will have to use your needlenose or small crescent very carefully to bend the outside arm of the cage slightly inward. But only slightly! This should be just enough to allow you once again to back out the high gear adjusting screw until the chain-cage contact while pedalling ends, and keep the chain from over-shooting the large sprocket while shifting.

e) If the chain rubs only at one spot when pedalling the problem is probably with your chain ring. Just as a wheel must remain 'true' to keep from rubbing against the brakes, a chain ring must be true or it will slap against the sides of the cage at certain spots. Back in Chapter One I suggested a five-pin crank over a three-pin for this very reason. Sometimes the chain ring bolts - the bolts which hold the front sprockets together - come loose and must be tightened. If you have done this and the wobble is still present, check to see that your bottom bracket assembly has not worked loose. While I have never

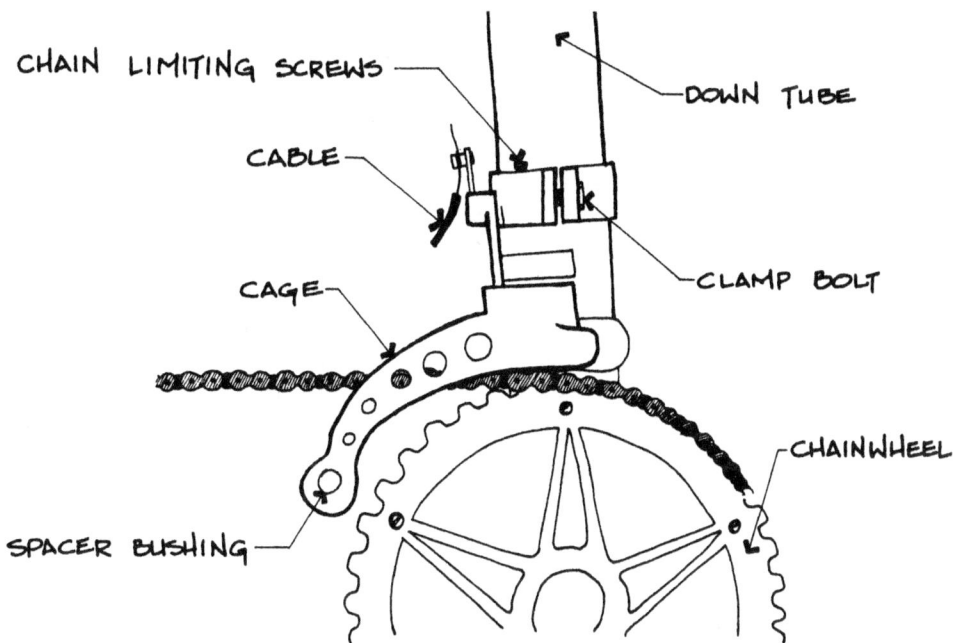

CHAIN LIMITING SCREWS
DOWN TUBE
CABLE
CLAMP BOLT
CAGE
SPACER BUSHING
CHAINWHEEL

FRONT DERAILLEUR

been troubled by an untrue chain ring which couldn't be corrected by one of these methods, you may. If you are on tour and have no other choice I would remove the sprockets and attempt, while praying fervently, to straighten them out with light hammering. But if you are at home, or in a town with a good cycle shop, I suggest you have a good shop mechanic help you.

j) If the chain rubs against the inside arm of the cage when you are pedalling in your smaller front sprocket, work with the low gear adjusting screw in the same manner as suggested above for high gears. With this problem you may have the chain falling off on the inside of the small sprocket. If so, bend the forward tip of the inside cage away from the derailleur housing. Again, do this very tenderly.

2. Your front derailleur refuses to budge when you tug at your shifter, or fails to return to its resting position when you release the cable tension by pushing the shifter handle forward. *The solution:*

a) The answer here is the same as with your rear derailleur - a frozen cable or a very dirty changer. Lubricate the cable and changer as discussed earlier. If the derailleur must be cleaned, a more thorough job can be done if it is removed from the bike. Removal and replacement suggestions follow.

b) Critical to the proper operation of a front derailleur is its north-south position on the seat tube. Most changers work best when the outside arm of the cage is about 1/8" above the teeth of the large sprocket. However, to save myself the time and trouble of finding the proper position when I replace my front derailleur to its home on the tube, I use the metal file of my Swiss Army Knife to nick the paint on the tube just above and below the derailleur mounting clamp. This allows me to slap the changer back on the bike in no time.

I realize that my suggestion to nick your paint purposefully probably horrifies you, especially if you have a brand new bike, or one which hasn't been battered much over time. For me personally, the beauty of my bike rests in its amazing combination of form and function, not in its paint job.

c) Once you have decided whether or not to mark your changer's location on the tube, loosen the cable anchor bolt and remove the cable.

d) Remove the bolt at the rear of the cage. Be sure to catch the small spacer brushing which rests between the cage arms, and the locknut and washer on the other side.

e) Remove the mounting clamp bolt which is furthest away from the derailleur body; loosen the other clamp bolt. Lift the derailleur from the bike.

j) Clean the changer in a pan of solvent. Brush the debris from springs and hard-to-reach areas with a toothbrush. Wipe clean and allow to dry.

g) Lubricate all springs and moving parts with oil. Remount the derailleur on the down tube; align the cage, and adjust high and low gear adjusting screws as necessary.

Chains

All motorists know how much better a car seems to run when it's been washed. Well, the same goes for a bike when the chain has just been cleaned and oiled. The interminable squeaks are gone, the derailleurs move quickly up and down the sprockets, and pedalling is as smooth as silk. All this being true, why on earth don't riders clean and lubricate their chains more often? The simple answer is that most do not know how to take the chain off their bikes, and cleaning a chain in place is almost impossible.

You will need a chain removal tool (also called a 'chain rivet remover') to take the chain apart. The tool costs about $3.25, and should be carried with you on tour - along with several extra links. This tool removes and replaces links, and frees 'frozen' links as well.

Take a close look at your chain and you will see a series of metal side plates with rollers set between them, and held together by rivets.

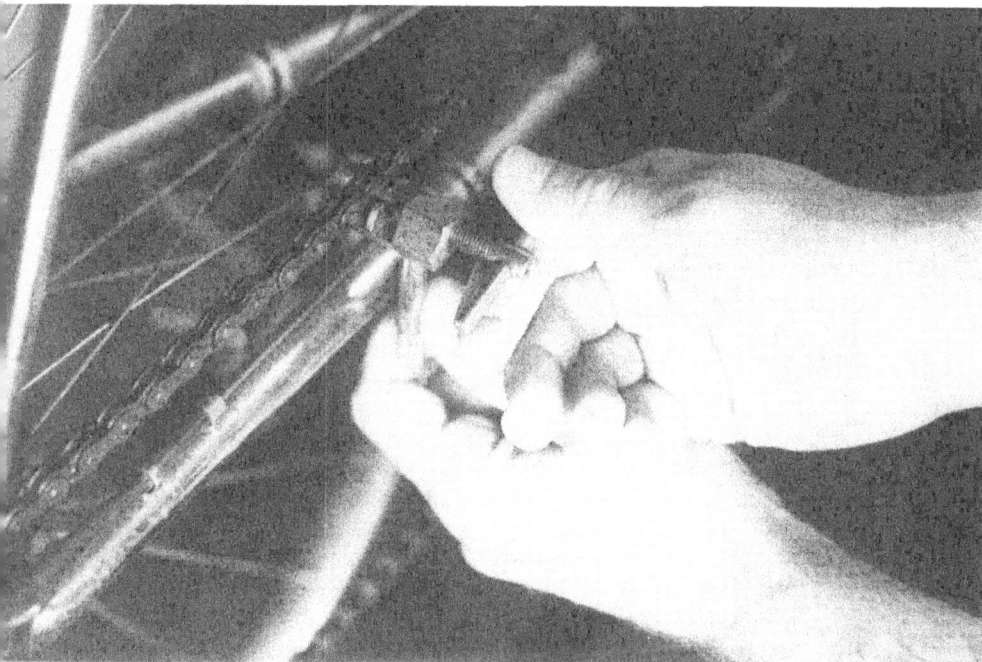

The plates overlap one another, and this presents us with one of the metal-upon-metal contacts in a chain which must be lubricated to prevent wear and noise. But the next point of contact is even more critical - the point where the rollers spin upon the rivets. This is where oil must be present to allow your chain its full life. a. When a link becomes frozen, it is often as a result of dryness, and makes itself known by jumping over teeth in the sprockets, or by causing the rear derailleur to jerk forward suddenly as it passes over the tension and jockey pulleys. Elevate your rear wheel and turn the pedals to find the culprit link, and when you do, coat it with a light oil and work the link with your fingers. This may free it. If it doesn't, you'll have to use the chain tool.

b. When viewed from the side, the chain tool looks like a wide 'U', with two shorter 'walls' of metal between. Place the tool in front of you with the handle to the left side. Twist the handle counter-clockwise to remove the rivet 'pin' from view. Now, take your chain, or preferably a few old links for practice first (many bike shops have old ones lying around which they'll give you), and place it over the first of these walls from the left. It will usually be somewhat wider than the right-hand wall. Notice, when you view your chain tool from the top, that these walls have an open space in the middle, and the chain roller rests in it, the 'plates' on either side of the wall. To free a frozen link it should be placed in just this manner on the left-hand wall. Turn the tool handle clockwise until the tool rivet pin touches the chain rivet. As you turn the handle more, notice how the plates move slightly farther apart. Most often only the slightest rivet adjustment is necessary to free the link. Be sure not to push the rivet flush with the side plate, for its length is such that it should extend slightly past the plates on both sides. If it is necessary to push the rivet flush to free the link, simply turn the chain over in the tool, and apply pressure against the opposite end of the rivet.

c. To remove the chain, it is necessary to drive a rivet out of one side plate, past the roller, leaving the rivet still held in place in the second side plate. This last part is the killer, and you should practice it a few times at home before having to do it on the road. (I have twice accidently driven the rivet completely free of the second plate; the first time I luckily had extra links around, the second time I did not. It took me a good half hour to wedge the free rivet back into the side plate, using the chaintool and my needle-nose pliers.) Place the chain over the right-hand wall of your chain tool, and turn the handle clockwise until the tool rivet pin touches the chain rivet. Some bike shop mechanics will tell you to then turn the handle six times without fear. This is supposed to place the rivet beyond the roller, but still in the far side plate. Perhaps they suggest this so nonchalantly because bike shops use a special pliers-like tool which in one quick squeeze of the handles pushes the rivet out to the exact desired spot. For me, it's touch and go past the fifth handle turn. Beyond that point I make a quarter-turn and pull on the chain to see if it will fall free, then another quarter-turn and another tug, and so on.

d. Once my chain is free from the bike I soak it in solvent, working all links and brushing the dirtiest plates with a wire brush. Then I suspend it from a nail to dry for a half-hour, and wipe away any remaining solvent at that time. To lubricate it, I place a single drop of light-weight oil on each roller, and rub the entire chain with an oiled cloth.

e. Replace the chain on the bike so that the extended rivet faces you; otherwise you'll be trying to use the chain tool backwards. When you have driven the rivet back through the roller and into the second plate you'll probably find the link to be stiff. If you do, place the link on the left-hand plate and free it, following the directions above.

Two common questions are: how do I know when I need a new chain: and, how do I know what length chain to buy? First, you need a new chain when you have an inch or more lateral play. Hold the chain in your hands, so that you are looking at the rollers, and move one hand to the right, the other to the left. An inch or more of side-play, if allowed to remain, will wear the metal teeth of the sprockets, the plastic teeth of the jockey and tension pulleys, and slap against the cage of your front derailleur.

Once you know that you do need another chain, count the number of links in your old one, and buy a new chain with exactly that number. But, should you need to fit a chain to your bike and for some reason you can't determine or trust the old length, follow this procedure. (It is not the easiest of all methods, but is in my opinion the most exact.) Put your new chain on the largest sprockets in front and rear. This should just about pull your derailleur cage until it is horizontal (your rear derailleur, that is), parallel with the chainstay. Give it some assistance by pulling the chain taut if need be, then lift the chain at the top of the chainwheel. You should have between V2 and 1 full link of extra chain at this point. Remove the excess links.

Finally: some general observations after fifteen years of dealing with chains.

1) Chains are responsible for 90% of the dirt on a bike, due to the attraction of road grit to all the oil on the links. For this reason I keep my chain just as dry as it will permit without beginning to squeak.

2) Chains are *not* responsible for that line of grease on the inside of your right pants leg - *you* are. The chain is where it is supposed to be; learn to mount and dismount your machine properly, and use pants clips at the cuff, and you'll stay out of its way.

3) I was on a ride to Yellowstone a while back when a fellow rider told me how he didn't use oil on his chain at all. He bought blocks of paraffin instead, melted them down in a coffee can, and dipped his chain. When it dried he put it on his bike. That was such a novel idea that I had to try it, though it didn't sound all that good to me mechanically. Bops and I did try it for a while, and found it great for keeping the bike free of grease. But we finally rejected it because of the hassle melting the paraffin, the relatively short time between required dippings, and the fact that we couldn't simply add a touch of oil when developing a squeak on the road.

4) Shimano has a new 'Link Lock' which acts as a no-tool-needed master link to take the chain apart. I tried it, and found it somewhat difficult to work with. When it comes dry and clean in its plastic bag it's easy to take apart and put back together, but after a few months on the road the grease build-up caused it to slip in my hands. Still, that would have been acceptable, but for the fact that I figure you have to carry a chain tool with you anyway, in case of a frozen link. So why drop $3.50 for a master link, when the chain tool is already in your pannier?

5) Check out any bike catalogue and you'll see many different kinds of chains - with specially formed side plates or cambered inner plates, beveled rivets and gold colors. Some are narrower, to fit a slim six-sprocket freewheel in place of the old five. Well, I just can't see all this for me. Somehow, it smacks at the universality of hiking. Where would I have been with one of these new chains had it broken down in India? These newcomers also require special chain tools, and cost more. And the gold-colored chain? - a real touch of Detroit.

This short guide to mechanics should keep you running smoothly. I haven't covered mounting instructions for generator lights, as the directions are included with the product. And I haven't mentioned how to attach luggage racks, partially for the same reason, but also because it is easier in this case to check out a bike shop floor model with mounted racks and follow it. (Each rack has its own particular attachment method.) Again, have patience in learning your machine. After all, it will be with you a lifetime.

Tools

In this section I will list the tools I have accumulated over the years, and which I find necessary or helpful in maintaining my bike. I will add current costs as averaged from three or more bicycle catalogues, or as determined locally in bike shops and hardware stores. I will indicate if I use the tool at home, carry it with me while commuting, or take it on tour. Finally, a list of the repairs or components for which these individual tools are necessary will be provided. (Where more than one tool will serve the purpose I will indicate my personal preference.)

1. *Crescent wrench* 6" - $6
   a) Uses - saddle, handlebars, wheel axle nuts, cottercrank, brakes, derailleurs, pedal removal
   b) Home, commuting, touring

2. *Crescent wrench* 4" - $4.50
   a) uses - Easier to use with brakes than 6" due to smaller size, same is true for derailleurs
   b) home, commuting

3. *Regular blade screwdriver* - overall length 6", blade tip 3/16" wide - $2
   a) Uses - tightening brake lever bolts on handlebars, handlebar end plugs, prying out dust caps over bearing cups, backing out pedal cones, derailleur adjustment
   b) home, commuting, touring

4. *Needle-nose pliers,* smallest available *with* side-cutters - $4
   a) Uses - pulling cables taut during replacement, cutting cables to length

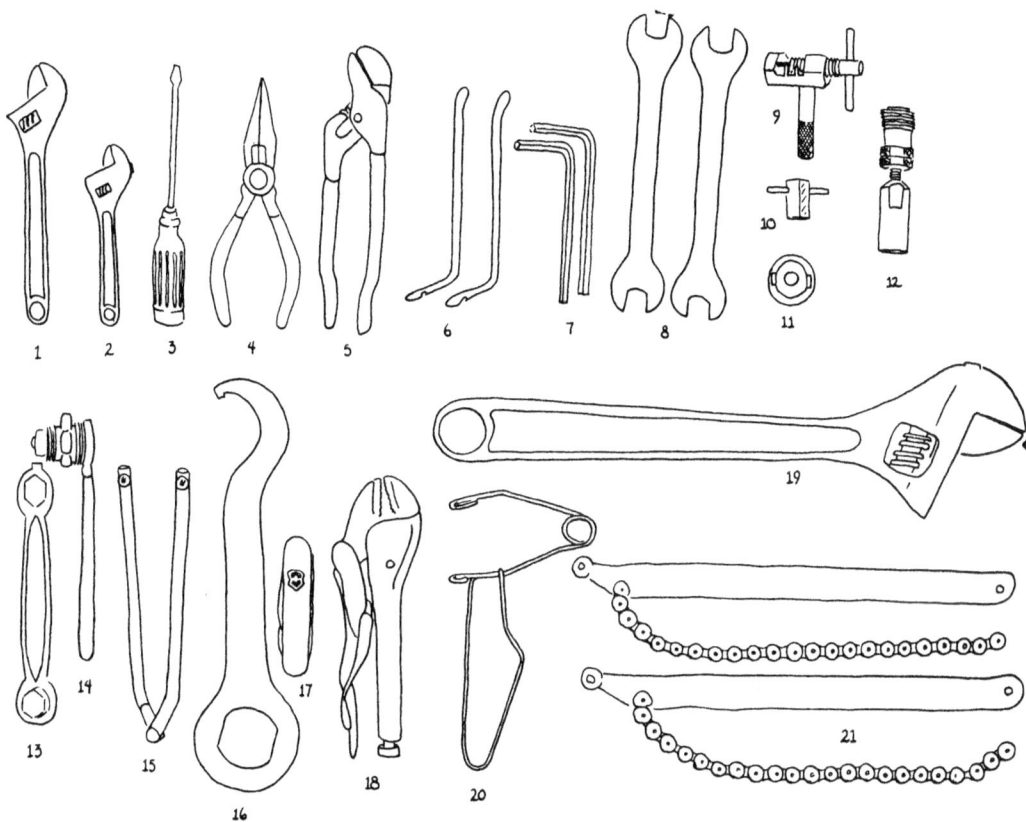

b) home, commuting, touring

5. *Channel locks 7" - $6.50*
   a) Uses - pedal dust caps, headset, freewheel removal on road
   b) home, commuting, touring

6. *Tire lexers-$1.50 for two.*
   a) Uses - fix flats
   b) home, commuting, touring

7. *Alien wrenches* - 75 cents apiece
   a) Uses - chain ring bolts, derailleur pivot bolts, crankarm dust
      caps some saddles and handlebars
   b) home. commuting, touring

8. *Cone wrenches* - two (13 & 14mm, 15 & 16mm) $2.50 per pair
   a) Uses - wheel bearing cone adjustment

b) home, commuting, touring

9. *Chain rivet tool* - $3.50
   a) Uses - chain removal and replacement, freeing frozen links
   b) home, commuting, touring

10. *Spoke nipple wrench 'T-type'* - 75 cents
    a) uses - spokes
    b) home, commuting, touring

11. *Freewheel tool* - Sun Tour $2, most others approx. $5
    a) Uses - freewheel removal
    b) home, commuting, touring

12. *Cotterless crank removal tool* - $4 to $8
    a) Uses - crank removal
    b) home, commuting, touring

13. *Universal cotterless crank wrench* - $11.50
    a) Uses - removal of crank arm fixing bolt (same as removal
       tool above, but made to fit all crank bolts. I have one
       only because of the many different bikes I service.)
    b) home

14. *Universal cotterless crank arm puller* - $10
    a) Uses - pulls crank arms (my reason for having this is same
       as above)
    b) home

15. *Universal adjustable cup tool* - $11.50
    a) Uses - adjustable crank bearing cup
    b) home

16. *Lock ring/headset tool* $7
    a) lock ring on adjustable crank bearing cup, raising and lower-
       ing headset
    b) home

17. *Swiss Army Knife* - Champion model $35
    a) Uses - metal file blade for protruding spoke heads, Phillips
       screwdriver for small screws holding LeTour generator light
       lens (has 13 additional blades/features)
    b) home, commuting, touring

18. Vise *grips* - $8

a) Uses - removing blips from wheel rims; hand-vise
when needed
b) home

19. Crescent *wrench* 15" - $14
a) Uses - removing freewheel, cotterless crank
b) home

20. *3rd hand brake tool*- $1.50
a) Uses - adjusting brakes
b) home

21. *Freewheel sprocket tools* - two, $6.95 pair
a) Uses - changing freewheel sprockets
b) home

The following items are not tools per se, but should be listed here because of their association with repair work at home.

1. *Bike tuning stand* - Persons $8, $4.50; Sun Tour $49.50
a) Uses - lifts rear wheel off the ground for adjusting
derailleurs, chain, crank arms
b) home

2. *Floor pump with air gauge* - $15
a) Uses - quicker, more convenient than the hand-held pump
carried on the road; the built-in air gauge is priceless - no
need to let air out while checking pressure with hand gauge
b) home

3. *Ball bearing grease* - there are several different kinds available,
and all come in a tube except for the kind I now use exclusively at
home - Drydene #4000. This comes in a plastic tub, and includes
a syringe applicator. It held up very well throughout the rain and
heat of last year's 3,000 mile Lewis and Clark trail, and costs
about $4 per pound, compared with $1.50 for a 3-ounce tube
of Phil Wood grease. Bike catalogues do not carry this Drydene
Lube, but you can send to this address for it:

JR Touring Cycles
P.O. Box 34127
Bethesda, MD 20034

4. *Oil* - again, several different kinds are available. Two which I have
used and liked are:

Sturmey Archer, 8.8 ounce can - $2.50
Cycle Pro, 7 ounce can - $1.30

5. *Wheel truing stand* - as I mentioned in the wheel truing mechanics

section, I have always trued my wheels without the aid of a stand, and still do not own one. However, Palo Alto catalogue has one which appears quite reasonable. I mention this because several of my friends trust a stand more than their thumbs and eyes for perfect alignment. $15

5. The Commuter's Checklist

Perhaps I should entitle this chapter 'This Commuter's Checklist', for no two riders I've ever known carry the same gear. I go a bit overboard with being prepared for all contingencies, while my wife is just the opposite. I carry almost the same tools when commuting five miles that I pack along on a worlder, though I've never needed most of them. Nevertheless, I'll list what I pack around the city, and you can choose as you wish.

On the Bike

1. Orange safety flag - thin, stiff, one-piece rod, $2.50 (may be hard to locate - I can't find them in catalogues. Try bike shops and department stores.)

2. Reflectors - at least in rear of pedals, and at end of rear rack.

3. LeTour generator light set - head and taillight both, $15

4. Water bottle filled with ammonia - bottle and cage $15

5. Luggage racks - front and rear; I use Blackburn, though they are expensive ($40 per pair approx.). However, I took the worlder with a Pletscher, which today costs $8.

6. Fenders - $12 per pair for black Bleumels. Colored Bleumels are $13; Esge (chrome-plated color) are $14.

7. Air pump - Zefal high pressure $12.50
8. Air pressure gauge - **$3**
9. Six extra spokes - taped in place behind the seat tube $1.1 also insure that the nipples do not screw off the shaft spokes by individually taping each nipple to the spoke.
10. Leather handlebar tape - **$6.50**
11. Compressed air horn - $4.25. This is so loud it hurts the ears, but is a great additiion to the handlebars for city riding. New vinyl-coated clamp at $1.90 is far superior to older metal bracket at $1.50.
12. Handlebar finger bell - $2.50.1 don't ride with one, but will if enough motorists become pedestrians and clog the roadsides a bit. Great for letting someone know you are present, without blasting them off their saddles with the compressed air horn. Perfect for college towns and cross-campus riding. (Lickton's catalogue)
13. Lock • my choice. Citadel - $25 (extra long shackle is $30)
14. Kickstand - alloy, $5
15. Rear view mirror - **$4**

Your daily commuting distance, the season of the year, and personal preference will determine which of the following items you decide to make a permanent part of your commuting bike bag. (An asterisk follows the items which I carry in my bag.) I have classified this commuting gear into the areas of:

a) tools
b) rain gear
c) cold weather gear
d) medical
e) miscellaneous

A. Tools
1. crescent wrench 6" - **$6** *
2. crescent wrench 4" - **$4.50** *
3. regular blade screwdriver 6" - **$2** *
4. needle-nose pliers - **$4** *
5. channel locks 7" - **$6.50** *
6. tire levers - $1.50 for two *
7. allen wrenches - 75 cents apiece *
8. cone wrenches - (2) $2.50 pair *
9. chain rivet tool - **$3.50** *
10. spoke wrench T-type - 75 cents *
11. freewheel tool - **$1.50** *
12. cotterless crank removal tool - **$4 - $8** *
13. Swiss Army Knife (Champion) - $35 *
14. tube patch kit - 75 cents *
15. spare tube - regular weight, $2 *
16. several links of chain - 50 cents *

17. extra brake pads (2) - $1 pair *
18. spare head and taillight bulb (1 each) - These I carry cushioned in cotton, held within a 35mm film cannister. $1.80 pair *
19. spare gear cable - 75 cents *
20. spare brake cable - 75 cents *

B. Rain gear
1. poncho- $18 *
2. rain chaps - $7 *
3. totes (rubber shoe covers) - $7.50 *
4. gaiters-$10 *
5. sunglasses - any glasses will help to keep the rain out of your eyes, but I suggest a safety strap to hold them on your head, and a good case so they won't be broken in your bike bag. *
6. glacier or snow goggles for night rains, when sunglasses would be too dark. $4.75 and up. *

C. Cold weather gear
1. jacket - $24 Long. light-weight, breathable; shell is 50% cotton, 50% polyester; lining is 35% cotton, 65% polyester. *
2. wool stocking cap - $4 *
3. wool sports cap - $8 up. I wear this on cool days, with the stocking cap in my bag as back-up if the evening breezes are colder. My sport cap is the English model with one snap in front - low profile to keep the wind from blowing it off. *
4. goggles - $4.75 and up. *
5. neck gaiter - $2.50 *
6. ski mask (Balaclava) - $2.50 - $7 *
7. gloves - $15 - $35 Buy the best your wallet allows. *
8. insulated underwear - $15. - $25 *
9. durable trousers - best I've found thus far are the Chouinard Double Seated Trail Pants, $32, from L.L. Bean. Chouinard also puts out great double seated shorts for about $20. *
10. socks - for warmth and durability I choose the 85% wool/1 5% nylon, 12" high - $4. *
11. light-weight boots - $45 - $90 *

D. Medical
1. Army style combat bandage - most people are unfamiliar with this excellent and inexpensive (49 cents) alternative to 4" x 4" compresses and gauze tape. Army surplus stores in your area might have them, or perhaps will order them for you. The bandage had very long cloth tails for tying around the body, thereby holding it firmly in place without the need for tape. I suggest this because of the nature

of most non-car-related bike accidents - a scraping away of the skin from contact with the road. Such a wound is beyond the band-aid, and more than what the usual first-aid kit carries in the line of thin cotton compresses and gauze. If you can't locate these I suggest several 4 x 4's and a long roll of gauze. *

2. Betadine solution swab-aids - $1. These are antiseptic-germicide pads which weigh little more than band-aids. They take the place of iodine in a bottle. *

3. band-aids - for all the minor cuts that come your way. 70 cents per box. *

E. Miscellaneous
1. spare shock cord - 50 cents *
2. trouser clips - (2) 75 cents a pair *
3. riding gloves - $9.25 pair *

Once again, allow me to stress the individuality of commuting gear. My wife has gotten along just fine with only rain gear, goggles, a spare tube, two tire spoons, a 6" crescent, needle-nose pliers, a brake cable and gear cable, and bike pump and lock - about half of what I carry. And as yet, she has never had to resort to that final bit of commuting gear she carries - a dime to call me if she breaks down. In five years she has never had to walk her bike home. So choose your equipment with care, and keep out from under cars on the road.

Note: I haven't mentioned helmets as a part of my commuting gear because I don't ride with one. I tried to wear one on tour in '66, but the discomfort was too great. Of course, a concussion or cracked skull is even less desirable, so if you don't mind the appearance and feel of a helmet you should wear one. (I've tried to talk Bopsy into wearing one in the past, but she has refused thus far.) All the bike catalogues at the back of the book carry helmets, but I suggest that you visit your bike shop and try a few on. I'd hate to see you drop $35 for something which isn't going to be used.

A second item I haven't mentioned is the bike rack for cars. I don't own one for obvious reasons, but I have looked them over and prefer the bumper-mounted carrier. I would buy the one which can be easily removed when not in use; the bumper brackets remain in place, the top part simply slips out and off the car. (holds 2 bikes - Bike Warehouse, $19.25)

And now, finally, we'll leave the city for the open road.

Part Three
Touring

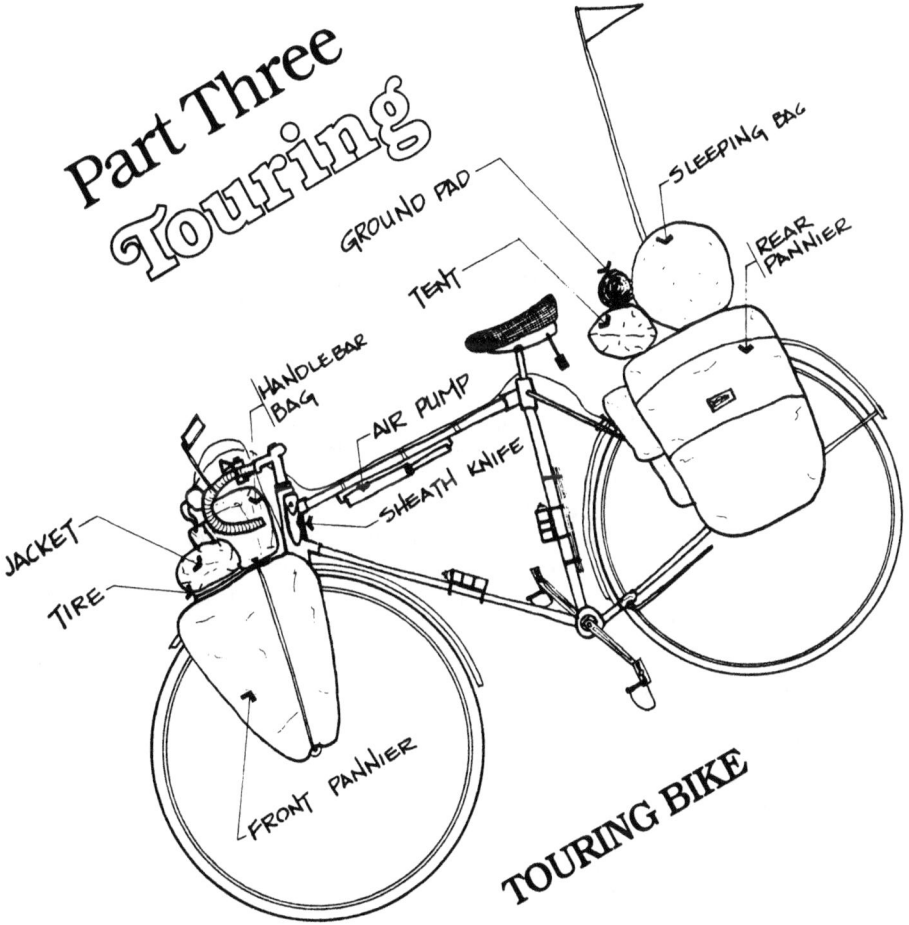

GROUND PAD

SLEEPING BAG

TENT

REAR PANNIER

HANDLEBAR BAG

AIR PUMP

SHEATH KNIFE

JACKET

TIRE

FRONT PANNIER

TOURING BIKE

I once heard the wife of a rock-climber say to a friend, "I just can't understand going *over* a mountain when you can go *around* it so much more easily." I really had to laugh at that. Her tone of voice and the expression on her face were almost identical to those of people who have quizzed me for fifteen years about my cycling. No doubt the lady's husband had tried to make her understand the rewards of climbing, as I have repeated the litany of reasons for touring the country by bike. But, finally, the talking has to stop, and *the feeling* must begin.

Touring by bicycle is for me the quintessential element in satisfying the age-old urge of mankind: discovery. Discovery of distant places is allowed by the remarkable mobility potential of a well-tuned bike on good roads. The discovery of different peoples is afforded not only by this mobility, but by the fact that hiking places the rider in a position where he must draw upon the population - water from farm wells, food from shops and stands along the way, road directions and permission from a hundred individuals whose common humanity is appealed to by the cyclist's request to unroll his sleeping bag behind a barn or garage. But these two forms of discovery are merely the most obvious - those which, when combined with a sense of adventure, made up the propellant force behind my first ride so long ago. It has been the countless other discoveries which have kept me in the saddle since.

Those other discoveries make up the indelible memories I carry of a hundred places in the past - rainstorms and headwinds, sharp temperature changes and baking summer heat, the differences between flowers and animals and even insects from one geographic region to another, the 'feel' of the topographical differences between the Midwest, the Great Plains and the Rockies - and a sense of camaraderie with those early explorers and settlers who likewise struggled across the land. Last summer I met a woman on our ride along the Columbia River who had ridden her single-speed bicycle from eastern Washington state to the coast - in 1939. She fascinated me with tales of headwinds and bad roads, of flat tires and good times with people she had met along the way. It had all remained so crystal clear to her, and I think the reason is in the experience which the mode of travel allows. Move across our nation inside an automobile and you see its beauty and expanse. Ride across it on a bike and you *are* a part of what you see, subject to the forces which have created the environment - from the scorching heat of the desert to the fears of life in a ghetto area as you pass through the large cities along your route.

It is this experiential element of cycling which allows for another of the fascinating discoveries of touring - the discovery of oneself. The physiological side of touring, that combination of physical preparation and psychological response to varied situations, grants the cyclist a terribly honest perception of himself. I know people who are forever going on a new diet 'as soon as the weekend (or holiday) is over', or others who work out only their jaw muscles continually talking of new exercise programs. But load up a bike with thirty pounds of gear. Pump it up a mountain or fifty miles across a plain, and all the self-deception about diets and physical fitness will be seen as just that.

Well, enough on the reasons for touring. If you aren't gung-ho to give it a try after commuting for a while, the experience probably isn't for you. But if those rides to and from work have merely whetted your appetite for more miles in the saddle, then read on. I'll give you all that I've learned while touring, and you can go from there.

6. Preparing for the Tour

My first suggestion in the discussion of preparedness for touring is simply - be realistic. My second suggestion, since number one is difficult if you haven't toured before, is - be prepared to change your mind as to what is and is not realistic, and then alter your plans accordingly. Now, this idea is not the stuff of metaphysics, nor for that matter is anything in cycling. But the simple dictum of 'be realistic' requires that the rider already know himself and his limitations, and few of us have ever searched those out. A number of riders over the years have asked my advice on touring, and I have found that ninety per cent of them accept my counsel readily - if it agrees with the plans they've already formed themselves. Now, I'm not talking about mechanics' tips or the clothing I find essential for a certain season. Where I find new riders going wrong most often is in the nature of the trip generally - the number of miles to cover daily, the monetary budget, training necessary before they ride, and whether a biker should bite off a journey solo the first time out.

Of course, few riders go wrong in all these areas, even on the first ride. Let's say a cyclist plans to cover eighty-five miles per day, carries funds equal to $7 a day, had ridden his bike every weekend and on four consecutive Sundays has racked up one hundred miles. How do we assess his preparation? The answer is that we can't, unless more information is supplied. Let me trace one possible scenario. First, our rider used service station maps to plan his route. So, what's wrong with that? The problem is that those maps tell only distances, and not the differences in terrain. Remember in Part Two when I discussed topographic maps, those which show the critically important element of elevation? Had our rider known to use topo maps he would have realized that whereas his practice Sunday rides were relatively flat, his intended tour route was quite hilly. Secondly, his vacation time being limited, he planned on 85 mpd (miles per day) every day, so as to see as much country as possible. But his training never included back-to-back rides of at least 85 miles; his work schedule had allowed him only one free day per week - Sunday. Finally, his money allowance was sufficient to carry him from starting point to destination and home again at $7 per diem, a reasonable sum if he ate only one meal per day in cafes, and, a point of critical importance, if he covered 85 miles each day. If, for some reason, he required two days to cover that distance, his money allowance was cut to $3.50 - a pretty meager sum at best. And we can see that even if the rider is fortunate enough to have no mechanical problems to slow him down, the unexpected difficulty in terrain and the soreness resulting from so many consecutive days in the saddle would surely chew away at his 85 mile average.

Our rider's downfall was in not allowing for a margin of error in his daily mileage, and the resultant effect on his per diem money supply. He tried to be realistic in his planning, but failed even in his training schedule by simple lack of experience. But, his tour need not have been ruined if he had followed my second suggestion - 'be prepared to change your mind as to what is or is not realistic, and then alter you plans accordingly'. If, once he realized his mistakes, he had shortened his tour by half or a third, he could still have enjoyed his journey and planned more wisely next time. If a tour is round-trip then a change in plans is easy; merely begin the homeward loop earlier. However, if the trip is one-way, with a return to home planned by bus or plane, the problem is greater. New riders seem to find it very difficult to admit an inability to keep up a daily mileage, and continue plugging away at it long after failure is obvious. Some, of course, manage to tighten their belts and gird their loins sufficiently to keep on schedule, even though they may be miserable. But this is I think the saddest case of all.

You can see how mistakes in planning feed upon one another, and why I always counsel a large margin for error. If the nature of the trip is more in the 'journey' category, such as a coast-to-coast ride, and the time element is crucial, then the margin for error is slight and the importance of training is stressed. I will discuss training in detail later, but first I want to cover the more general topic of the different 'kinds' of tours. This decision will, after all, determine necessary training, expenses, daily mileages, clothing lists and all the other particulars which follow in the next few pages.

Deciding on the Kind of Tour

Basically, there are three kinds of tours; camping, motel or hostel, and a combination of camping and motels.

1. Camping tours - On this kind of tour a rider saves the expense of motels, but must carry his home (sleeping bag and tent), with him. The added weight cuts into the daily mileage, but offers the freedom of choosing where to bed down each night, thus freeing the cyclist from the schedule of having to make it to a certain motel each day.

2. Motel or hostel - Most Americans are unfamiliar with hostels (inexpensive overnight lodgings primarily for persons on hiking and cycling trips), but do know of the many forms of motels in this country -motor lodges, Motel 8's. Best Western, etcetera. Although there is an organization called the *AYH* (American Youth Hostel), most of these lodgings exist along either coast. (See appendix for addresses or AYH.) If you travel abroad you have a real treat in store for yourself, as many of the hostels are located in quaint or historic buildings. I have slept in interesting hostels in London, Austria, Jerusalem, and on a island in the Nile. Back home, a Motel 8 may be far less romantic, but believe me it is just as welcome at the end of a long day's ride. (Having spent many nights in both motels and hostels, I find it interesting that the isolation of travel by automobile is reflected in the motel, whereas the more common experience of pedalling or hiking is reflected in the hostel practice of meals taken together in a dining hall, and often in shared sleeping quarters. That may seem to be forcing camaraderie, but I have met some fascinating people in hostels abroad.)

3. Combination camping/motel - This is the form of tour I have taken for the past five years; i.e., since my wife decided that this was the kind of tour for us. Always before I had prided myself in the varied sleeping arrangements I could find, unrolling my bag in abandoned ice houses, garages, barns, jails and warehouses. There-has also a perverse pleasure in seeing just how much money I could keep from spending on a ride, with ninety per cent of it going for food. Well, all that has changed, and now I find myself every third night or so re-clining on a soft mattress after a hot shower, watching the news on television. Not that I'm griping, mind you, but I am happy I've had both kinds of rides.

Which kind of trip you finally choose will be dictated by your wallet, the area you wish to travel, and naturally your personal inclination toward the outdoors. I know riders who love a day of pedalling through the countryside, but would not begin to consider sleeping on the ground; for them the perfect day's ride ends in a comfortable motel lobby. Others I know are equally conscientious in their avoidance of motels. But to fall into either strict category is to narrow greatly your options of areas to travel. Those who must stay indoors will be forced to omit huge expanses of lovely countryside which still do not sport Hiltons and Ramada Inns. And those earthly hold-overs of a decade given to herb tea and vegetarian diets, who think it 'impure' to partake of a 'bourgeois' motel, will find camping out a bit harrowing in the industrial centers of large and mid-sized cities.

Again, hiking offers the sanity of the middle road. Just as using a bike for commuting and shopping can save the gasoline and finances for an occasional weekend drive, so too does touring by bike allow such a financial saving that a nice night in a motel is affordable. (This should serve to reduce the motels' 'impurity' to the second group, for I have often noted that their categorization of 'bourgeois' applied primarily to institutions they could not afford.) As to convincing the non-camper type to go a night in a tent to see if he might like it, the chances are much better for success if the non-camper is the tired biker at day's end, and still a long ten miles from town. I'm confident that once both groups have had a taste of the other tour style they will opt for motel/camping combination rides in the future.

Alright, we're clear on that point - if you have chosen the combination tour your area of riding is limitless. You have decided on the kind of ride you'll take; the next step is in planning the route. Perhaps you have thought that a certain area you have heard or read about would be great to tour, or that it would be fun to pedal into another state to visit friends or family. If visiting someone nearby, you probably have a good idea of the distances and terrain, but you will not already know the best route for bikes. And if you've chosen a region you've only heard of, your need for information is even greater. Let me help you in gathering that knowledge.

Researching the Tour Area

I have told you of my first cross-country tour, planned with an insurance company atlas which devoted one page to each state. I would have been better off with service station maps. But today I do not feel prepared until I've exhausted the following sources.

1. Begin with an atlas or large wall map which provides the geographic relationship of your tour area to the nation as a whole. (I am assuming, since this is your first tour. That you have chosen an area in the U.S.) Seeing your area in this context should provide you with a general orientation as to weather, population, and terrain. It will also enable you to begin paying attention to your intended area when the national weather report is given on the news.

2. Pick up the most recent service station maps available, and choose a tentative route which stays away from interstate and other major highways. Many stations charge a nominal fee for these maps, which is understandable, especially when you bypass their gas pumps on your bike. If you know someone who belongs to an automobile association you might ask them to pick up some free maps for you.

3. Review the discussion in Part Two of topographic maps, then send away for copies of the ones you'll need. Service station maps have a scale of about one inch to every 18 miles, but you can obtain topo maps which are detailed to the point of one inch equalling only 2,000 feet. This is the scale I have suggested for commuting, but for obvious reasons such maps are impractical for touring. The topo maps I suggest are the 1:250,000 Series (1 " = about 4 miles); the area shown on the map will be 107 square miles. These are good maps to pack with you on a ride, though the number you carry will be determined by the intended length of your tour. On long tours it may be convenient for you to mail a packet of maps ahead, to a post office in a town you are sure you'll be riding through. Choose a small town, so you won't waste an hour trying to find the correct post office in a big city, and mail the package to yourself, marking the envelope 'General Delivery' (Post Restante if abroad). The normal policy is to hold a letter for ten days before returning it to the sender; you will have to extend this period by writing on the envelope "Please hold until July 15, 1981," or whatever date you feel is a good week or so past the latest time of your intended arrival. For major journeys I would extend this period to more than a month, as any number of problems may detain you. However, you must insure that the post office will comply with your wishes by sending a letter of your intentions to the town's postmaster.

The 1:250,000 Series map is fine for touring, but I like to plan the tour in detail using the 1:62,500 Series (1" = about 1 mile) for the areas I'm most interested in, and the 1:24,000 Series (1" = 2,000') for the larger towns in which I plan to spend a couple of days sightseeing. Carefully studying these maps with friends before your ride will enable you to form a clear idea of terrain, and thus will provide the opportunity to alter routes *before* you find yourself staring at an unexpected range of mountains.

4. Write to the state department of transportation to inquire about roads restricted to bikes, and ask them for any guidance they might feel would be helpful concerning your intended route (early snowfalls in the mountains, heavy traffic, etcetera-). Your reference librarian will help you obtain the necessary addresses.

5. Write to the Chambers of Commerce in the larger towns on your route, outline your plans and ask them for general information on the area. Request the name and address of any local bicycle club, for if you are lucky enough to be touring an area which does have one, you'll have lucked into a gold mine of information. Chambers of Commerce encourage tourism, and if the state has a specific department of tourism, they will request information for you from that source or send you the address.

6. Write to the national League of American Wheelmen organization, requesting addresses of local chapters in your tour area. Fellow bikers can always give the most appropriate touring information.

7. I have found the general information on weather conditions received from Chambers of Commerce and state departments of transportation and tourism much more helpful than the specific data on maximum/minimum temperatures and monthly precipitation averages available from the U.S. Weather Bureau. Besides, you'll be prepared for all weather variances once we've packed your panniers.

8. Finally, obtain the address of the state historical society from the Chamber of Commerce, and write to them requesting information of historic trails you might be crossing on your route. Also, request the names of books on state and county histories. You will be amazed at how much more interesting an area can be when you know how a particular mountain range or pass got its name, or that your modern-day road follows an ancient Indian trail.

This may appear a very time-consuming bit of letter writing, but it can all be packed off in a couple hours if you simply develop a form-letter type explanatory paragraph, and follow it with the specific request of that particular office. Besides, the wealth of information you'll gain will be considerable payment for two hours' work. You will find any number of interesting sights you would have missed by researching early, and you'll be able to plan more realistically for daily mileages. Many times I have heard riders say "If I had known the country had so much to see I would have planned another week!" Don't shortchange yourself - do your homework ahead of time. And now we are ready for the next vitally important step in preparing for a tour.

Physical Conditioning

Perhaps the greatest number of questions which come my way about touring concern the topic of getting into shape. Most do not believe me when I answer that a modicum of fitness, a well-tuned and properly loaded bike, and a willingness to spend hours in the saddle are all the requirements necessary to pedal across your city, or around the world. My words are usually met with smiles and skepticism, but they are nevertheless true. It is difficult for people to imagine how very easy it is to tour by bike, for they place pedalling in the same category as tennis and jogging in the need for a physical outlay of energy, or think it is similar to backpacking as far as discomfort. Touring is none of these things. It is what you will make of it - an endurance run of one to two hundred miles each day, a highly mobile but more human-paced eighty mile per day trip, or a leisurely and civilized thirty-five to fifty mile daily tour. Herculean strength is unnecessary; your physical prowess must only equal the nature of the tour you plan for yourself.

In Part Two I spoke of the areas of your body which will be sore following your first few days on a bike. You will remember that I warned you of soreness in neck, arms, hands, back, stomach, bottom and legs. Recalling this now should help to illustrate that hiking in general, and touring in particular, requires physical fitness throughout, not the enormous calf and thigh muscles most non-bikers expect. Therefore, in designing a physical conditioning program to prepare for touring you may feel confident that any and all exercise helps. And this is true from simply walking to the best of all training possible - riding your loaded bike.

If you are already commuting by bicycle you are halfway through the necessary training, for you have worked through some of the soreness which can ruin a short tour, and cause you to lose valuable time at the beginning of a long ride. However, for those of you who plan to go from not owning a bike in early spring to touring by the summer, I will outline a simple regimen which should have you in shape by June. Do not forget that this is only the most general program, and that each person must tailor it to himself as his body (and spirit) requires. (A detailed explanation of the program follows the chart.)

12 Week Training Program
(for 35 to 50 mpd tours)

Week one
1. calisthenics - 5 reps each (daily)
2. riding - 2 to 3 miles easy terrain (daily)
3. walking - V2 to 1 mile brisk pace (if you don't have your bike yet)

Week two
1. calisthenics - 5 reps each (daily)
2. riding - 5 miles easy terrain (daily)

3. jogging - short distances interspersed with walking (daily)

Week three
1. calisthenics - 7 reps each, less rest time between exercises (daily)
2. riding - 5 miles easy terrain (daily)
3. jogging - slightly longer distances, less walking between (daily)

Week four
same as week three

Week five
1. calisthenics - 10 reps each, no rest between exercises (every other day)
2. riding - 10 miles easy terrain
3. jogging - same distance as week four, but no walking (jogging and calisthenics on same day, riding on alternate days)

Week six
1. calisthenics and jogging same as week five (3 days)
2. riding - 10 miles moderately hilly terrain, or 15 miles flat country (4 days per week, alternate days)

Week seven
same as week six

Week eight
1. calisthenics and jogging may continue as time permits, but concentration is upon riding for last 5 weeks
2. riding - 10 to 15 miles easy terrain, with half of expected tour weight (daily)

Week nine
1. riding - half expected tour weight, 10 to 15 miles hilly terrain (daily)

Week ten
1. riding - all expected tour weight, 10 miles hilly terrain (daily)

Week eleven
1. riding - all tour weight, 20 miles hilly terrain (daily if time permits, at least alternate days)
2. riding - weekend overnight trip, all tour weight, 35 miles on both days

Week twelve

1. riding - all tour weight, 20 miles hilly terrain (daily if time permits, at least alternate days)

2. riding - weekend overnight trip, all tour weight, 50 miles on both days

The thought of spring and warm weather has excited you to consider a bike tour in June; it is the first week in March and you have ordered your bike and panniers, but they won't arrive for a couple of weeks. Can you begin training without your bike? The answer is yes, and with only twelve weeks to go you should begin immediately. Do so by critically assessing your present physical condition; can you walk up a flight of stairs without losing your breath? Can you do twenty push-ups or a half-dozen sit-ups (with knees bent) without back pain, and without feeling like someone slugged you in the stomach? Finally, can you jog a half-mile at a slow pace without being thoroughly winded? Chances are if you haven't been on a physical fitness program, and if your job is sedentary in nature, you won't be able to do these things. But don't despair. The human body is an amazing adaptive apparatus, and will quickly accept new requirements if you give it a chance to do so gradually.

The key to good cycling is endurance, and your training should reflect this. Five sets of twenty push-ups will be of greater value than two sets of fifty; a slow jog of a mile is better for you than running the 220 yard dash. Why? Because the nature of cycle touring calls for endurance rather than quick, short bursts of great energy separated by periods of rest. Before your bike arrives, and continuing afterward, you should decide upon a daily calisthenic program. But for your own sake start off easily - five jumping jacks, 5 toe-touchers (knees locked), 5 stretchers (legs spread wide, hands on hips, upper torso movement to front, sides and back while bending at the waist), 5 push-ups, 5 sit-ups. The first few times you'll have to rest between exercises, after a while (a week or so) you'll be able to do them almost without rests between. When you move to this point increase the repetitions of each exercise. If five reps are too much to begin with, cut back to 3 and work from there. You must always remember that you are exercising for yourself, not to satisfy some cold statistical chart of physical data. To be beneficial your exercises should bring on a degree of breathlessness, but not to the point of wheezing and gasping for air. Increase your repetitions as your body tells you it is able to do so. But be honest with yourself - don't let a recalcitrant spirit hold you back, or a heady desire for quick progress push you past the boundary of caution.

If you have your bike for this first week you should be riding 2 to 3 miles daily over easy terrain. If you are still bike-less, however, substitute brisk walks of $^1/_2$ to 1 mile in length.

After a week of exercises begin a regimen of slow jogging. (Running shoes are expensive, but well worth the money.) This will greatly increase your wind, and start to develop your legs. (The calisthenics concentrated upon upper torso and arm muscles. I did not recommend deep knee bends, as most sports physicians today feel they are hard on the knees.) When I taught physical education to junior high school boys I found the most successful method of building their endurance to be two weeks of run/walks - running an 1/8 mile, walking an eighth, running again, then walking once more. This took them twice around a quarter mile track for 1/2 mile total. In the third week I changed this to running a quarter mile, walking an eighth, running another quarter, and walking the last eighth, for a total of 3/4 of a mile. Two weeks of this brought them to running two half-miles separated by walking to an eighth, and finally, when six full weeks had passed, the students were up to one full mile without rests.

Most of us do not have tracks available for training, but we do have city blocks. Many cities in the East and Midwest count twelve blocks to the mile; Salt Lake has seven to the mile, others vary between. A call to your local highway department or street commissioner should provide you with the information, and if not merely pace off a block, figuring each step at 1 yard (440 yards = VA mile). Begin with a jog of a half-block, then walk a half, another jog and walk, and then see how you feel. Hopefully, you will not require a cab to take you home. If you feel strong try jogging a whole block the next day with a half-block rest between, and so on up to a mile. Distances beyond a mile are excellent for increasing endurance, but remember that the best exercise for local touring is cycling, not running or lifting weights or doing isometrics. If you have the time for daily jogs of more than a mile *and* frequent riding, then do so. But do not allow any other form of physical preparation cut into your time in the saddle.

Some of you may have access to weights, but I hesitate recommending any regimen for as diverse an audience as those who may be realistically considering touring. Therefore, let me say that if you already train with weights you can definitely put them to your advantage, but that if you don't you should be extremely cautious in beginning weight training. Many such classes seem to stress exercises which produce bulk - large muscle groupings designed for quick bursts of maximum power output - *not* endurance. Thus I suggest a trip to your public library instead, and a perusal of books on weights. You will find programs designed to prevent development of large musculature, and to enhance endurance. Basically, this is made possible by increasing the number of repetitions of an exercise, while using only light weight on your bar and dumbbells.

Personally, I train with weights because they can provide me with a hard workout in far less time than would be required without them. For example, thirty sit-ups while holding a ten pound weight behind my head takes only half the time of the 60 to 90 sit-ups which would be required without weights for the same result. Also, weights can exercise certain muscle groupings which are difficult to reach through calisthenics or jogging alone. These muscles can be put to work through sports, but long ago I realized that any physical fitness program necessitating the presence of other people would be far too infrequent for my needs. The human body's physiology is such that 'weekend athletes' become prime users of Ben Gay and ace bandages. (Try using your brain only two days of the week and see how sluggish it becomes.) My weight program stresses exercise for arms, shoulders, neck, chest, stomach and back muscles. Jogging, and my riding to and from work keep the legs in shape. I alternate weight lifting and jogging day-to-day, unless my schedule is such that both seem to be required. Oddly enough, the greater the pressures upon my time and my psyche from a job, the greater the need for exercise as a respite. Any teacher who doesn't commute by bike or in some other fashion exercise daily is staring insanity in the face.

Okay, you are up to ten reps of calisthenics and a quarter mile jog per day after a month. You've had your bike a week, spending that time adjusting handlebar and saddle height, and getting used to the 'feel' of the machine. (If you haven't had your bike until now you can still catch up, so don't be disheartened when the bike shop is slow in getting it ready.)

Begin with an unloaded bike. By that I do not mean to leave your tools and tire pump at home - always ride with them. But wait a bit before you start hauling the 25 to 30 pounds of gear you'll be carrying in the summer. If you already are jogging a quarter-mile, begin with a 5 to 10 mile ride over easy terrain; if you have had your bike all along, then you will start your calisthenics, jogging, and cycling within the same week. In this case ride 2 to 3 miles over easy terrain once each day for a week, then move up to 5 miles daily. One more week of this and daily rides of 10 miles over easy terrain should work you through the inevitable sore spots. Now, I realize a problem with time may arise at this point, for a 10 mile ride will require about an hour. The best way to solve this difficulty is to ride to and from work; if, however, this solution is impractical for you then I suggest a 10 mile ride every other day, with your calisthenics and jogging on the alternate days. Later in the training period, you may decide to skip the jogging completely, but until then I recommend the running to develop your wind.

In the sixth week, when you begin tackling hills, use your arms to help you 'pull' your way up, and concentrate upon the ankling technique discussed earlier. If you don't have enough time available for the 10 mile rides then pace yourself at a bit faster then normal riding speed for the number of miles you do have time for. What is 'normal' speed? Whatever pace you are comfortable with on the road, and can maintain throughout the day, will be normal for you. Invariably a tour with six people will find six different cycling paces, and you should deal with this fact before the trip begins, by riding together often.

As indicated in the Training Program Chart, the last five weeks are spent primarily in the saddle, with partially or fully loaded panniers. (See below for help in loading your bike bags, and some pointers on becoming accustomed to riding with them.) Don't become discouraged when those areas of your body which you thought impervious to pain after the first difficult weeks begin to hurt anew, for you'll work through this within a few days. Pedalling a loaded bike taxes muscles far more than merely riding additional miles unloaded. Be prepared for early difficulties in handling and steering; these will subside along with an impression of the general 'clumsiness' of a loaded touring machine. It is all-important that these few weeks be spent riding loaded - that you do not wait until the trip begins and merely try to 'learn as you go'.

Preparing for Group Tours

If you are planning a solo ride your training is a personal matter, but if you'll be cycling with others your physical condition is no longer just your concern. This is true for two reasons. First, the weakest member determines the day's progress. Due to time schedules and return-trip transportation plans, a daily average must be discussed, and agreed upon as a group. Such a discussion early on in preparation for the tour will make clear to all riders exactly what kind of trip is envisioned. One member may have in mind an easy, carefree ride; another may wish to cover more ground per day. This must be settled early in the training period, so that all members work toward a common goal.

The second reason why an individual's physical condition is a matter of mutual concern lies in the psychological effect upon others which one tired, sore rider can have. It is important to understand that to enjoy continual fifty mile days one must be able to pedal even farther - that a cyclist bone-weary and completely without strength in reserve following such a ride will be poor company for a group. 'Successful' when it conies to a ride cannot mean merely reaching the destination; bike touring which turns to drudgery negates the very reason for hiking.

You may think this so obvious that it needn't be discussed, that all members would naturally train together to insure proper physical preparation. And this is the case when each individual has the group, and not just himself, in mind. But, let me warn you to make sure you are planning a ride with people sufficiently mature to judge their own capabilities, and either train to extend them, or drop out of the trip for the benefit of all.

I once made the mistake of giving up on my demands for group training before a particularly arduous tour, and paid a heavy price for it. We had travelled by bus to the starting point, and on that first morning straddled our bikes and prepared to mount up. But then came trouble. One rider, trying to pedal out of the parking lot, could not control her bike. Here we were, a thousand miles from home and three times that from our destination, at the end of a six month period of preparation for two months of touring through some of the most difficult terrain in North America, and one member of the group had not ridden a single mile with her bike fully loaded for travel. Sick at heart for this inauspicious beginning, we dismounted and watched as the rider circled the lot for forty minutes, trying to accustom herself to the weight. But, if I was sick at watching this and all it portended for the next few weeks, it was nothing compared to my emotions when she finally wheeled back to us, unsteadily dismounted and said, "Well, I can stay on the bike now. I just can't shift gears."

Finally, don't hope to catch up in physical condition with the rest of the group on tour, if you have begun as far behind as the unfortunately true example above. This is because the others riders will of course increase in strength at a relative pace, and the one sore cyclist will become even more distraught when he sees himself becoming stronger, but still unable to maintain the group's pace. Decide together on the kind of tour, research the area thoroughly, and train as a team. Such preparations will insure a happy ride.

7. Touring Equipment

By this point you have purchased your bike, equipped it along the guidelines in Part One, decided upon the kind of tour you'll take, researched your route, and have begun your training program. Now you are ready to consider the items which will make up your home, bed, wardrobe and resource center on tour. I'll give you my equipment list, but you'll have to tailor it for yourself, of course. And don't worry about hurting my feeling in doing so; my wife scoffs at half the stuff I carry in my saddlebars. As with commuting, the range of 'necessary' equipment is as broad as the differences between cyclists. Allow me to prove this point with the following story.

Back in 1965 my buddy and I parked our heavily-loaded 3-speeds outside a restaurant, next to two gleaming bicycles which sported only fenders and a rear view mirror. Shortly after seating ourselves at the counter two gentlemen in their sixties approached us. "You young fellas on tour?" they asked. "Yes sir," we replied. "We're heading up to Canada." "Well, we're on tour also," they announced proudly. "Those are our bikes out there. Been gone two weeks now."

This amazed me, but I was polite enough not to comment on their age. Instead I asked a question about their mounts.

"But, where is all your gear? Your bikes don't have a thing on them."

The men smiled contentedly, as one unbuttoned his left breast pocket and extracted a fold-up toothbrush.

"This, and our checkbooks," he said with assurance, "are all the luggage we need."

I haven't made up an equipment list in the last fifteen years without thinking of them. Those hardy men were on one end of the spectrum as far as gear on tour goes, but I am very close to the opposite extreme. Where you fall between these two poles depends upon the modifications which the nature of your journey, and pure personal preference, require.

As with the kind of bike to buy, and the make-up of the 'commuter's bag', no list of mine should keep you from wisely 'individualizing' your touring equipment. However, there are good reasons why I carry each and every item on my list, and thousands of road miles have given me a wealth of experience to assist in my compilation. Hoping not to tire you, I will provide explanations for the items where I believe it will be helpful.

Before I begin, let me try to anticipate a question about climate, and how it affects my equipment list. Surprisingly, my gear changes very little due to seasons, for even my summer rides often cross mountain passes, requiring cold weather gear. I will explain where changes are made for seasonal touring, and give reasons why in the notes following each item. A final checklist without annotation will appear at the end to serve as a more simple guide once you have read all the explanations.

My touring equipment list is divided into the following eight categories:

A. Clothing
B. Foul and cold weather gear
C. Shelter and bedding
D. Medical supplies
E. Personal
F. Miscellaneous
G. Tools
H. Bike parts

A. Clothing

1. T-shirts (3) - all bright colors, but not white. White T-shirts only look good when very clean, and yours will be gray before long -besides, even if they have a pocket you'll still look like you're wearing underwear in public. So that doesn't bother you? Well, how *you* feel about it isn't the point; it doesn't make sense, especially while on tour and periodically in need of assistance, to give offense to people a bit more conservative than you. Another point - all your clothes must be able to be washed at once, together. Mix a pair of dirty riding shorts and a white T-shirt in a washer and you'll come out looking like an old Easter egg.

Why three shirts? While on tour any clothing directly next to your body should be washed daily - socks, underwear, T-shirts. Having three allows one to be worn, one to be drying (strapped on top your sleeping bag on the rear carrier - held in place by shock cords), and one as back-up in your pannier for those occasional nights when you can't wash your day's wear.

The shirts should be of good quality to last the tour, one size larger than you normally take to provide ease of movement, and should have long tails to remain inside your riding shorts when bent over the handlebars. Make sure that *all* your clothing is washed and machine-dried several times before your trip, to check on shrinkage. Why machine-dried? Because there will be times when you can't rely on the sun for that service. And why bright colors? For two reasons: you'll be seen more easily on the road, and you'll look a lot better on your slides.

2. Long-sleeve shirt (1) - permanent press, full cut, long tail and extra long sleeves to protect the wrists when arms are extended in riding position. The material should not be heavy, for the purpose is

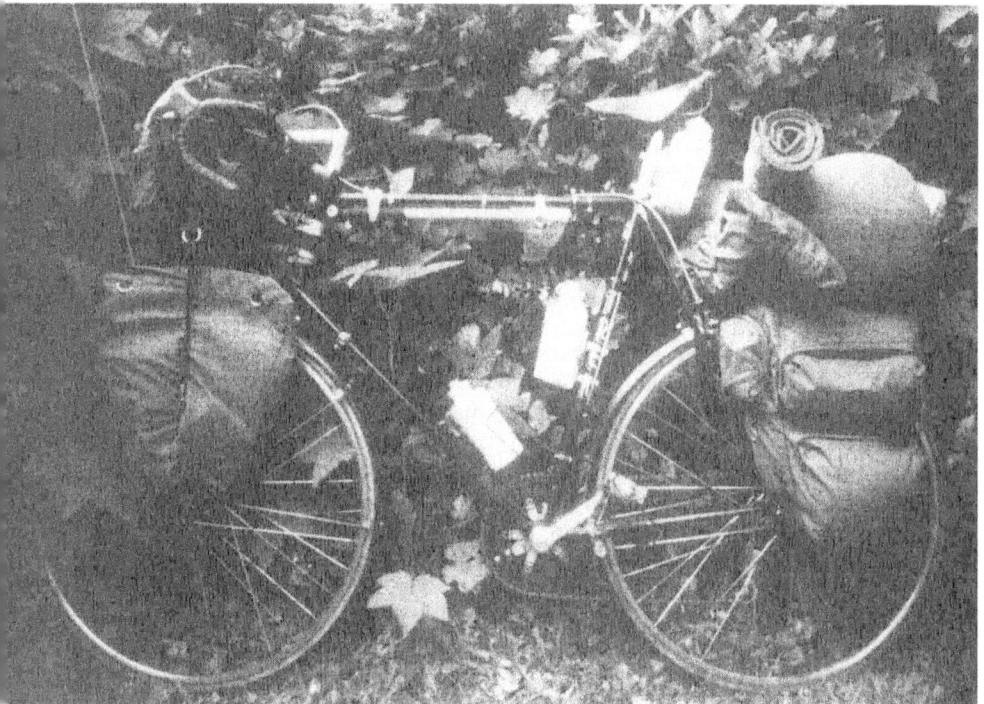

not warmth (other clothing is available for that). Light material will compress nicely in the pannier, and will be sufficient to provide arm protection from mosquitoes. (It would be difficult to wear a heavy shirt for this purpose on a warm night.) As I mentioned when discussing clothing for commuting, turtle neck shirts are too warm for my use. Even the kind with the short zipper neck will not allow you to control your body temperature as will a shirt which buttons completely down the front. I don't ride in this shirt often, and generally try to keep it clean for wearing in towns and motel lobbies.

3. Riding shorts (2) - highly durable material, belt loops, pockets. The belt loops assist in tying the rain chaps in place, and a belt is preferable due to the considerable weight loss sometimes experienced on tour. Pockets are a good idea so as not to leave your wallet on your bike in towns, and as a place to hold the handkerchief which is often needed in cold weather. The special riding shorts with sewn-in chamois bottoms do not have pockets or belt loops. These shorts are also quite expensive, and advertise that underwear need not be worn. You might expect this weight and space savings to be reason enough for their purchase, but I prefer to wear undershorts which can be changed daily, and washed easily. The special riding shorts are generally hotter due to the nylon or polyester fabric used, and the older styles were tight-fitting around the thighs, allowing no air to circulate. New touring shorts which promise to stretch in all directions and are loose-fitting at the thigh can be purchased by catalogue (see appendix for address), but still more expensive than those I use. Check out the surplus stores for khaki pants, which I've picked up for $4 a pair and cut off for riding. No corduroy, but the heavy cotton duck will wear forever.

4. Belt (1) - Army type, slip buckle. This will allow for the inches you might lose around the waist; it can be used as an emergency sling or tourniquet, or can double as a shock cord.

5. Undershorts (3) - you'll probably choose jockey shorts if the weather is such that you might not have to ride in long pants. If so, be sure to have loose-fitting shorts which won't chafe you.

6. Long pants (1 pair if you are on a summer, fall or spring tour, 2 if a winter tour; when taking 2 cut riding shorts to 1 pair) - durable material again; which means no corduroy. Blue jean material wears well, but is very heavy and bulky, weighs a great deal when wet, and takes forever to dry. Preferably permanent press. Be sure legs are long enough to still cover ankles when pedalling. (Review discussion of clothing in Part Two)

7. Gym shorts (1) - these will serve as a pair of riding shorts in a pinch, and are good for swimming.

8. Insulated underwear (1 pair, separate top and bottom) - reread what I have said about them in Part Two. They should be some color other than white, for the top will sometimes serve as a second long-sleeve shirt or as a sweater. Be very careful about the shrinkage problem, especially as they must be machine dryable for the tour. Long-sleeves, tail, and legs to remain in socks.

9. Protogs (1 pair leggings) - these beauties are well worth the high cost of $ 16 for anyone who has ever ridden fall or spring tours. (I carry mine in summer also.) With these 100% washable wool leggings you can start the cool morning ride in shorts, for the black leggings slip right over your sock and warm the area between mid-thigh and ankle. When the afternoon sun appears merely roll down each legging and put them in your pannier. Protog has arm warmers also, and a complete line of washable wool products, but I have only found a need for their leggings.

10. Socks (3 pairs) - height and material will depend upon the season, though in summer I usually ride without socks. In winter I choose 12" high, 85% wool, 15% nylon.

11. Riding shoes (1 pair) - Wayne and I wore low-quarter construction shoes on the 'worlder', but the most satisfied I have ever been on tour was in my Brooks running shoes. They were still enough so as not to give arch pain (the reason why tennis shoes, and most running shoes, are our for riding), and very comfortable on and off the bike. Some riders have complained about the damage done to running shoes by toe clips, and although I've not had these problems, several manufacturers have come out with special touring shoes. The Italian Deto Pietro TD is a real gem, but the upper construction is suede and therefore would not dry as quickly as others. Besides, the shoe costs $40, compared to $13 for the canvas (and washable) Bata Biker riding shoes. Both are available through Bikecology. For winter tours I switch to light-weight boots, described in Part Two.

12. Camp moccasins (1 pair) - lightweight, nice protection for socks or bare feet around camp.

13. Bandanas (2) - right colors, for you may wish to use them as signal flags at some point. A bandana can provide just the right degree of warmth around the neck on days not cold enough to require the neck gaiter. When wet, it can be just as cooling. Any number of uses will become evident when you replace the white handkerchief with a bandana.

14. Riding gloves (1 pair) - to keep you from losing all feeling in third and fourth fingers on long tours, as happened to Wayne and me in '74. Several weeks of near constant pressure with the heels of ungloved hands against the bars appears to affect nerves running to these fingers, though the numbing sensation passes within days when off the bike.

15. Baseball cap (1) - for those sunny, baking days when hair alone is insufficient protection. (Especially important for those of us whose foreheads reach increasingly higher each year.)

B. Foul and cold weather

1. boots (1 pair) - see Part Two for comments.

2. neck gaiter (1) - see Part Two for comments.

3. wool cap (1) - this goes on all tours with me, summers included. For very cold winter tours I suggest the Balaclava 'helmet', wool headgear which fits like a regular wool watchcap when folded up, but pulls down into a ski-mask type face protector. The neck is sufficiently long to tuck under the coat collar of neck gaiter. (L.L. Bean, $6.75)

4. light-weight jacket (1) - as described in Part Two.

5. gloves (1 pair) - cloth for summer tour, warmest gloves you can afford for other seasons. Read my notes on gloves in Part Two.

6. poncho (1) - I carry a poncho and rain chaps for all tours. Refer to Part Two for comments on poncho style.

7. rain chaps (1 pair) - Part Two.

8. rainsuits (1) - two-piece good material with air vents, bright color, long legs and sleeves. I sometimes prefer a full rainsuit to poncho and chaps on winter tours, when staying dry is critical, not just a matter of comfort. More in Part Two.

9. raincap (1) - a detachable hood is fine. This should accompany you on all season tours, and should have a drawstring attached in such a manner so as to facilitate pulling it tightly about the face; too often a loose raincap or hood without drawstring will ride forward on the head and block all peripheral vision. Choose a bright color.

10. rain boots (1 pair) - for all tours. Part Two.

11. goggles (1 pair) - Part Two.

12. down or fiber-fill jacket (1) - this jacket will take the place of the large sweater so many riders try to carry on their first tour. The jacket can be compressed into a very small waterproof stuff sack and carried outside the panniers; sweaters are very bulky, weigh more, and fail to keep you warm. Perfect for the occasional cold summer evening at high altitudes, when combined with insulated underwear and long-sleeve shirt it should provide all the warmth you'll need during winter days. On some bitterly cold nights in the Rockies I have slept wearing my down jacket inside my sleeping bag.

C. Shelter and bedding

Only three pieces of equipment appear under this heading - tent, sleeping bag, and ground pad - but all three are of critical importance and therefore require a few words.

1. Tent (1) - it is true that a cyclist can tour without a tent. I have done so. But I will never do it again, even for the great savings in weight. My reason is that I cannot have an enjoyable day, no matter what the scenery, if I've been sleepless the night before. And only a tent can provide protection from rain and mosquitoes - two of the three greatest challenges to spending a comfortable night under the stars. The third problem - cold - is dealt with primarily by the sleeping bag, though here again a tent is helpful in reducing windchill.

You will have to decide on what size tent to buy according to your personal situation; if you are married, or single but plan to tour with friends, you'll probably choose the two-man size. If you know for sure that you'll be touring alone I would opt for the Pocket Hotel, a two pound tent with floor and mosquito netting, which folds up as small as your down jacket. It is made of gore-tex, a material I discussed in Part Two, and has had good test results by cyclists in some of the outdoor magazines. It is 7V2 feet in height, 3 feet in width at the shoulders, and 2 feet high at the head. This should provide ample room for one. I have not tried it myself, and therefore hesitate to endorse it fully, but the Early Winter's catalogue offers a one-month full refund field test to all buyers. My concern would be condensation inside the tent once snow builds up on the outside. Buy you could check this yourself by buying it in the winter, and sending it back if you are dissatisfied. Similar to the Pocket Hotel ($149) is the Bivi-Sack by SierraWest (Recreational Equipment Incorporated catalogue, $125), the Super Bivy 1 (Yak Works, $122), and the Eastern Mountain Sports Pak Foam Super Bivvy Sak 1 ($110).

Before we go to the two-man tents I should mention the Early Winters Sleep Inn, an 18 ounce gore-tex sleeping bag cover, which makes your bag approximately 10 degrees F warmer, and which is designed to be used as a bivy sack as well. (By the way, if the word 'bivy' is bothering you don't hope to find it in Webster's, for it isn't there. 'Bivy' comes from 'bivouac' meaning "a temporary encampment in the open, with only tents or improvised shelter." Therefore, a 'bivy', 'bivvy', or 'bivi' sack is one which provides the shelter of a tent.) The Sleep Inn has mosquito netting, a strong tent floor material, and a gore-tex top for water resistance. I took a winter ride in Southern Utah last year with two friends who used these sacks on nights when the temperature fell into the twenties; in the morning they shook off the frost and climbed out warm and dry. I haven't seen them used in a downpour or heavy snow, however, and therefore still have some reservations. But, again. Early Winters offers the sack on a 30 day full refund trial basis.

You will have to spend a long time with your buddy or mate when choosing the right 2-man tent, for there are many kinds offering individual advantages. I suggest you send away for all the appropriate catalogues and, if possible, visit a store in your town which has floor models you can actually crawl around in. For me, a tent must be bug-proof, rain-proof, wind-proof, easy to set up and take down, and not unreasonably expensive. Outside of the Army I have owned two tents, both of which satisfied all these requirements. You might ask why I bought a second tent if the first met all the prerequisites. The answer is that I bought the first while single, and when I married, I found that my wife had another requirement which my Gerry pup tent could not meet - ample room inside to change clothes.

Some friends suggested the tent they had seen while backpacking in Yosemite - the 4 pound 11 ounce Sierra Designs Starflight ($165). We bought one, used it on the Lewis and Clark Expedition, and found it excellent in almost all ways. My single complaint, not shared by my wife, is the color - yellow and blue. My old Gerry was green, and I purchased it in that color for a reason. With a green tent you are able, in most areas of the world, to camp out rather inconspicuously in the woods or jungle. I thought there might be times on our world ride when we would appreciate blending into the landscape, and in my opinion the same is true in the States. Another problem I have with flamboyant tent colors is what they do to the landscape - to me they appear as bright billboards in an otherwise natural setting.

Nevertheless, the Starflight withstood the Pacific Northwest rain, the Midwest insect population, and a windstorm in Iowa which nearly scared me into reconsidering my agnosticism. When skies were clear we kept the rain fly in the bag, which allowed up to watch the stars through the spacious screened window in the tent roof. (This window also allowed welcome breezes to pass more easily through the tent than would only a single door opening.) When rain threatened we put the fly in place, and stayed snug and dry. In case you are unfamiliar with tents let me explain the construction. Taking our Starflight as an example, the floor is a heavy coated waterproof nylon, extending up the tent sides twelve inches to assist in keeping out floods. The tent walls (12" from the ground and all the way up to the top) are made of uncoated, breathable rip-stop nylon. This fabric allows the moisture in exhaled air to pass out of the tent, and not to collect on the tent roof in the form of condensation. But what keeps the rain from passing through this fabric? That is the job of the tent fly, a hardy, coated waterproof nylon sheet. (The fly must not rest next to the tent wall. for this will trap the moisture inside and cause condensation to form.)

You will notice that the gore-tex Pocket Hotel does not have a fly, and yet is waterproof. This is possible due to the special features of this material, where the thousands of microscopic holes in the fabric are too small to allow raindrops in, but large enough to let exhaled water vapor molecules pass out.

The Starflight is double-stitched along lines of stress, and enjoys 8 to 10 stitches per inch throughout. The resultant strength is attested to by the guarantee - if any stitching fails it will be repaired at no charge. Poles and pegs are of strong but light aluminum, and all fits into a stuff sack measuring 25 inches long and 7 inches around. Best of all from my wife's standpoint is its uncommon height - 54" -allowing even tall men to sit up inside without difficulty. (Tent length is 96", greatest width 64", width at either end 42".)

The Starflight is an A-frame style, just like the backyard pup tents of old. But you'll see in the catalogue that other styles are available -square, dome, arch-bow, et cetera. Most are too heavy or bulky for bikes (I would try my best to stay under 5 pounds), but some are elegantly shaped and should be considered. Among these: the FasTent Instant Shelter (4 pounds, $146) by Yak Works, the Light Dimension (3 ³/₄ pounds, $284), the Winterlight (4V2 pounds. $347), and the Omnipotent (5Y4 pounds, $295), all by Early Winters. If you are still trying to catch your breath after reading the prices of the last three tents you'll understand another reason for my choice of the Starflight. However, considering the costs of motels even the most expensive tent I've mentioned could be purchased for ten nights' lodging costs. And good tents last! My old Gerry has had seven years of rough use on all kinds of terrain and in all climates. Even my students have used it - the ultimate test - and it hasn't dropped a stitch yet.

Note: Practice setting up your tent several times before your tour, and, while it is up, coat the seams with 'seam sealant' or 'seallock'. This product comes in liquid or light paste from ($2 - 2.50), and prevents water from seeping inside your tent through the tiny stitching holes. You won't have to take any sealant with you on tour, as a liberal application will usually last several seasons. But I would (especially on tours abroad) carry 6" of rip-stop repair tape (V2 ounce, 35 cents). This is tape similar to that used by sailmakers, and is excellent for field repair of rips in tents, tent flys, your poncho, or any nylon product.

Note: After much use a tent zipper (with metal slide and hard plastic interlocking teeth) can fail to function. A quick and often successful repair can be accomplished by gently squeezing either side of the metal slide closer to the plastic teeth. Use your small channel locks or needle-nose pliers to do so.

2. Sleeping bag (1) - sifting your way through the terminology and choices to be made concerning sleeping bags is almost as difficult as choosing the right components and pannier system for your bike. Therefore, it might serve to make the topic more understand-able if I define some of the terms before I begin a discussion of the various bags.

a. shape: there are four basic shapes to sleeping bags - rectangular, semi-rectangular, modified mummy, and mummy.

Rectangular bags are most like your bed at home, squared off at either end and the least efficient of the four shapes as far as retaining body heat. This is due to the air space between your body and the bag around you - the greater the space, the more your body must work to heat the area. Although some comfort results from the relative freedom of movement inside the bag, the weight of these bags and their poor insulating qualities make them unacceptable for touring.

Semi-rectangular bags are squared-off at the top and rounded at the base, reducing somewhat the inefficient air space. Again, however, the squared-off top does a poor job of retaining the heated air which your body has burned up so many calories to produce. Thus, a poor choice for possible cold nights on tour.

The next bag, the modified mummy, is my choice for cycling. Un-like the first two, this bag is contoured to the body's shape, closes snugly about the shoulders, and has a pillow-type hood which on very cold nights can be drawn up around the head so that only the face is exposed. (On winter tours I use a ski-mask or balaclava to reduce even this exposure.) However, unlike the fourth bag (the mummy, which feels like a cocoon and looks like its Egyptian namesake), the modified mummy is just roomy enough inside to keep you from feel-ing like you're sleeping in a mail slot. It also has sufficient room to keep the next day's clothes inside with you, so that they'll be warm for the next morning. (Climbing out of a toasty sleeping bag and into ice-cold clothes at dawn is not my favorite way to begin a day's ride.)

b. insulation: sleepings bags do not provide any warmth of their own - their function is to retain the heat which you produce by burning calories while you sleep. (Cyclists on winter rides will be warmer if they eat meat, cheese, and carbohydrates for dinner - as fuel with which to stroke the furnace for the night. This point will seem clearer once we understand the definition of the word calorie - a quantity of food able to produce "the amount of heat needed to raise the temperature of one gram of water one degree centigrade.") At home, sleeping in a heated room, two forces work to provide a warm night's sleep - the heat of the body, and the heat in the room provided by that other furnace which runs on gas, oil, wood or coal, rather than food. Remove or greatly reduce the heat from the second furnace and we reach for another blanket, to trap even more of our body's own heat. Completely remove any heat source other than the body and you immediately see the need for either a great number of blankcts, or a single layer with superb insulating qualities. Naturally, in a sleeping bag there is but one layer, and this is where the importance *of the fill* -the insulating material of which the bag is made - comes into play.

Without question, the warmest, lightest insulator around for sleeping bags is Down, the "soft, fine feathers" from geese and ducks. It provides the greatest *loft*, the height of the insulating material inside the bag (and very important for warmth - the greater the loft the greater the heat retention). At the same time a Down bag is more compressable than any other. With the greatest warmth, lightest weight and smallest size, Down might appear at first to be the only choice. But there are other factors which must be considered.

First, Down is very expensive. Secondly, its miraculous insulating ability is lost if the bag becomes wet. And, third, Down bags must be expensively dry-cleaned, or, in a very time-consuming manner soaked in a tub with special cleanser (to aid in restoring its loft when dry), spun in a machine washer, hung outside for several days, and then tossed about in a machine dryer with a tennis shoe to help reduce Down 'clumping'.

Wayne and I carried good Down bags on our 'worlder', and it was one of our worst planning mistakes. We found it impossible to keep our gear totally dry in some climates, and were soaked through several times. This made for some very cold nights, and for many disagreeable ones, as dry cleaning was impossible in most areas, and washing by hand too lengthy a process to bother with. I remember an afternoon in Israel when we hung our bags over a clothesline and tried to break up the clumps with broom handles. But it didn't work, and thousands of miles later we paid dearly for our mistake when our battered sleeping rolls, having shed feathers on several continents, were all we had to keep us warm on our race to reach home by Christmas.

Obviously, the touring cyclist who expects moisture to be a problem needs a different insulator than Down - one which will keep him warm even when wet, and which is simple to launder. Luckily, these qualities do exist in the man-made synthetic fibers called *PolarGuard*, *Hollofil*, and *Hollowbond*, Bags made of these fibers also cost far less than down, but as with all things there are disadvantages. Synthetic bags weigh about one-third more, and cannot be compressed into as small a stuff sack as Down. (Stuff sacks are the bags into which you literally stuff your sleeping bag each morning. Don't try to fold your bag nicely to pack it away, for it won't fit. Also, make sure your stuff sack is waterproof before the tour.) Of the three synthetic fibers, PolarGuard has received the most praise, and surely receives mine. I have used my PolarGuard bag since 75 and have no complaints. Cleaning is simple - pop it into a washer on low temperature, then into a dryer also set at low heat. Inexpensive, convenient, and warm even when wet - a good bag for hiking.

Early Winters offers a fourth synthetic choice, which they claim provides "all the advantages of down and synthetics - and none of the drawbacks of either!" I'll provide the specs later, but for now let me just add that their secret lies in placing what they call a "Silver Lining" between layers of PolarGuard. This lining, developed for the space program, is designed to block "almost 100% of radiant heat loss." To understand this we must go beyond the explanation provided by Early Winters.

When you are inside your sleeping bag, heat is lost in two ways -convection and radiation. Convective heat loss refers to the actual movement of heated air from around your skin, through the bag, and escaping outside. This is the same heat loss which you retard by pulling a blanket or sleeping bag of Down or synthetic over you. Radiant heat loss has to do with the emission of energy in the form of electromagnetic waves; the emitted energy from the surface of any body increases greatly as the temperature of that surface increases. When these electromagnetic energy waves reach a surface which is not transparent to them, that surface absorbs the energy - and this is what the Silver Lining is said to do.

When you begin shopping around you'll see estimates of the *comfort rating* of each bag. Don't assume that your comfort and their comfort are the same, however; its like the E.P.A. mileage ratings for new cars. And just a couple more terms now. *Fill weight* refers only to the weight of the insulator material inside; *total weight* includes the lining, zipper, drawstring, snaps and fill. *Shoulder girth* refers to the important fit around the shoulder. Most of us needn't worry about this figure being too small for comfort, but you football players might want to throw a tape around yourself to see if you need a larger bag. As to length, each manufacturer has its own standard on 'regular' and 'long' bags, so be sure to check that you won't hang out of one end. Finally, the warmth of a bag is affected by its construction as well as its material, and you will find the terms 'sideblock baffles', 'slant-tube', and 'sequential - differential' in the spec charts. My honest feeling here is that your mental health and my blood pressure will best be served by relying on the 'comfort rating' to help you gauge the bag's warmth, and not by a lengthy explanation of construction.

Personally, I look for the following in a bag:

1. PolarGuard fill

2. 2-way zipper (to open from top and bottom)

3. zipper which allows for bag to be zipped together with a second bag

4. modified mummy shape

5. lightest weight possible in bag with comfort rating of approx. +15 degrees F

6. waterproof stuffsack

7. reasonable cost

I suggest you take a close look at the following bags, which satisfy some or all of the options I prefer. (All weight and cost data are those of the large or long bag - cyclists 5' 10" tall or less will find their bags a bit lighter and less expensive.

Name	Catalogue	Fill	Shape
Tuolomne	Sierra Designs	PolarGuard	Mod. Mummy
(4 lbs. 7 oz., 15 degrees F minimum, $99)			
Silver Lining	Early Winters	PolarGuard	Mod. Mummy
(3 lbs. 7 oz., 10 degrees F, $170)		Silver Lining	
REI Pasayten	REI	PolarGuard	Mod. Mummy
(3 lbs. 7 oz., 15 degrees F, $103)			
EMS Franconia	EMS	PolarGuard	Mod. Mummy
(5 lbs. 2 oz. 5 degrees F, $95)			
EMS Berkshire	EMS	PolarGuard	Mod. Mummy
(4 lbs. 9 oz. 20 degrees F, $80)			

3. Ground pad (1) - the third and last of our items under the heading "Shelter and Bedding," and as important to a good night's rest as both the tent and sleeping bag. As I mentioned earlier, ground pads are necessary to insulate the body from the cold ground, assist in keeping moisture from developing on the tent floor, help reduce the compression of the 'loft' of insulation in the underside of the bag, and provide an element of mattress-like comfort which, while slight, will be appreciated after a few hours on the hard earth.

Fortunately, choosing a pad is a far simpler process than selecting either a tent or bag. Basically the choice is between an air mattress or *foam pad*. If you decide on the pad, you must then choose between closed *cell* and *open cell* Once this is done you will determine the thickness of your pad by the climate you'll be touring in, and finally the *length*. Now, let's discuss the choices.

a) Air mattress or foam pad? - generally, the former is chosen for its sleeping comfort, the latter for its insulation abilities. While air mattresses are compact and very light, they also must be blown up each night and can develop troublesome leaks. On tours I try my best to reduce the number of possible problems, and thus free myself from fears of ruptured seams by choosing the more bulky, somewhat heavier, but considerably warmer foam pad.

b) Open or closed cell foam pad? - again the choice is between comfort and insulation. Open cell is soft, but requires three times the thickness to equal the warmth of closed cell pads. And, the deciding factor for me, closed cell is completely unaffected by water.

c) How thick a pad? - various manufacturers differ slightly on the insulating capability of closed cell pads, but generally suggest that ¼" thickness on cold ground is ample protection to 20 degrees F, 3/8" thickness to 5 degrees F. and ½" thickness to -10 degrees F. For open cell pads a 2" thickness is necessary for the coldest rating. My choice here is the ¼" thickness closed cell (even for dead of winter tours), primarily because of the difference in weight. The Ensolite closed cell 56" long pad weight nine ounces if ¼" thick, but fourteen ounces if 3/8" thick. And five ounces is a lot of weight on tour.

d) What length pad? - although a full length pad is nice protection from the cold ground, due to the weight factor I suggest a three-quarter length. On cold nights when I don't want my legs to touch the tent floor I place a half-empty pannier with clothes inside at the end of the pad, and rest my legs on it.

My good friend and cycling companion Bob Welsh would think this section incomplete if I didn't mention the ground pad/air mattress combination with which he tours. Called the Therm-A-Rest, it is self-inflating, comfortable, warm, and waterproof. But it also weighs three times as much as my Ensolite pad, and costs $34, compared with $6 for mine. When you check the stores and catalogues for closed cell pads you'll find, among others, the brands Frelen XL, Volarfoam, and Ensolite. The Volarfoam is not quite as durable as Ensolite; the Frelen XL I have found only in ½" thickness, and therefore I choose the Ensolite, Type ML, closed cell pad - *W x* 21" x 56", weighing nine ounces and costing $6.

D. Medical Supplies

1. Sunshade (1) - if you have trained long and hard for your tour, you might not need this, but take it along anyway. Although I gradually acclimate myself to the sun each spring to lessen the chances of burning, I still pack a 4 ounce bottle of lotion, for seldom during training have I been exposed for several days in a row.

One area to pay particular attention to is the thin band of skin just above your waistline in back. This area is exposed only when leaning over in riding position, and therefore is often missed by the sun until the tour.

2. Aspirin (20) - carried in a small prescription bottle.

3. Snakebite kit (1) contains small suction cups. scalpel, tourniquet, antiseptic, and directions on what to do if bitten. Few people are actually bitten, even for all the fears and horror stories. And even fewer people read the directions before it's too late. $2.50.

4. Desitin (1 tube) - this excellent cream antiseptic for small cuts is also the best antidote I've found for the terrible pain of sunburn, and for the even more difficult itching which accompanies it. I recall a ride out West in '66 when my buddy and I baked going across Kansas. Not knowing of such analgesic creams as Desitin we spread vaseline over our blisters, and even concocted a baking soda paste - all to no avail.

5. Hydrogen peroxide (1) - I carry a small bottle as a mild antiseptic to wash out cuts and scrapes. It will foam when you pour it on a wound, but don't worry - it doesn't burn like alcohol and iodine. (Be sure to pack it in the tiny brown bottle it comes in, or in a bottle which will permit no light inside. Sunlight breaks down the chemicals in this solution.)

6« Band-aids (10) - carry these in a waterproof container (I curl mine into a plastic 35mm film cannister).

7. Butterfly closure bandages (6) - I carry several of these in various sizes, also packed in a film canister. Butterflies are small bandages designed to serve as temporary stitches by holding both edges of a wound together. They look much like band-aids, but have the shape which gives them their name. You shouldn't have any trouble finding them in a drugstore, but ask your family doctor for a few if you do, or visit the neighborhood medical center.

8. Combat bandages (1) - accidents on bikes usually result in large skinned areas of legs, arms, and hands. Especially when touring in summer, the thought of bare skin sliding along on the pavement should bring on a critical assessment of the 'First Aid Kit' which so many people carry in their cars. My greatest criticism of these inexpensive kits is the tiny quantity of gauze which they provide. Therefore, I supplement my gauze supply with an Army combat bandage (49 cents) available in some surplus stores. This bandage measures 6" x 3" x 3/4" thick, and is adequate for very large wounds. If you can't find these you should carry extra gauze compresses as a supplement.

9. Gauze compress pads 4" X4" (4 to 8) - these plain gauze pads are very thin and thus not as absorbent as the combat bandage mentioned above. If I have the large bandage with me, I carry 4 of the gauze pads, 8 if I do not. These pads are packaged only in paper, and must be kept dry; I carry mine in a zip-lock baggie.

10. Gauze (1 roll, 2" x 20 yds.) -1 sometimes use gauze alone as a bandage for a small cut, wrapping it around several times and then cutting the last 2 linear inches down the middle, so as to tie it in place.

When using the corn presses I tie them in place with long strips of gauze. A zip-lock plastic bag will keep the roll dry.

11. Ace bandage (1) - for minor sprains and weak joints. My wife wears one around both knees in cool weather, for the added warmth appears to keep them from hurting.

12. Tube petroleum jelly (1) - excellent for chafed areas, chapped lips.

13. Benadryl a prescription - only antihistamine used as an antidote to allergic reactions to plants, insects, et cetera. Most of you who are highly allergic to insect bites already know to carry this, but it is possible to have an allergic reaction to something which had not bothered you a great deal before. Consult your physician about this drug.

14. Insect repellent - I carry a single 2 ounce no-leak plastic bottle. Before you buy, read the list of active and inert ingredients. The 'inert' ingredients do nothing to keep the bugs away, and yet in most repellents make up ^ of the bottle. The active ingredient to look for is Diethyl-metatoluamide. If you can find the old Army Jungle Juice' repellent in surplus stores, buy it - for it has 75% active ingredients. (REI catalogue has this for 95 cents if you have no luck locally, and Early Winters catalogue offers a 1 ounce bottle of Muskol repellent for $3, which they claim is justified by the 100% active ingredients. At this price I'd stick with REI.)

15. Water purification tablets (1 bottle) - one to two tablets according to the condition of the water you are drinking. (We used 2 per water bottle in India, though generally one per quart is sufficient.)

16. Moleskin - a great 'second skin' prohibitor of on-coming blisters. Buy it at your drugstore, but carry it wound inside a film canister or zip-locked in a plastic bag. And don't wait until the blister appears to treat it; you'll have to go the Desitin and band-aid route if you do.

E. Personal

1. Towel (1) - thin hand towel, not a bulky bath towel.

2. Washcloth (1) - the proper use of a washcloth is what makes it possible to dry off completely with only a hand towel. Following a shower or bath wring out the washcloth completely and dry with it as you would a towel. Usually the washcloth will be saturated after just the upper torso; wring it out again and dry your lower half. Now you can finish drying off with your towel. Not only do you save on weight and room in your panniers, but you end up with only a damp towel, not one which is soaked.

3. Soap (1 bar) -1 generally carry one small bar of Lava, which is abrasive enough to use when I hand wash my clothing. However, if the ride will include much camping in wilderness areas I pack a biodegradable soap like Dr. Bronner's. ($1 for a 4 ounce bottle) Another advantage with Dr. Bronner's is that the soap can be used as a shampoo.

4. Soap dish (1) - because touring cyclists prefer to tour on roads they seldom stray far from civilization. However, on the outside chance that you do, and because I try my best to choose items which I can also use while back-packing, buy an aluminum soap dish (49 cents) - in a real pinch it can be used as a signal mirror.

5. Toothbrush (1)

6. Toothbrush case (1)

7. Tooth powder (1) - unlike paste you'll never find it gumming up the sides of your bike bags. Pack it, or a combination of salt and baking soda, in a small waterproof plastic bottle.

8. Comb (1)

9. Toilet paper - I carry about 20 sheets in a plastic zip-lock plastic bag.

10. Deodorant (1) - a fellow graduate student used to extoll the virtues of life without this product, but I'm afraid he failed to convince me of the advantage inherent in a more odoriferous existence. When touring, it is difficult to wash and change clothes as often as at home, even though the need is greater. Thus, a bit of assistance on the scent side is helpful. (It also makes practical sense on tour, when you must deal with people who might think it more 'natural' for man to strive for cleanliness.)

11. Shampoo -1 only carry this if I don't have Dr. Bronner's.

12. Tube goop (1) - a small tube of this or other waterless hand cleaner and grease remover is just the thing when you drop your chain between towns. This way you won't have to use your drinking water to clean up.

13. Nail brush (1) - this may sound extravagant after making choices of items based upon differences of a half-ounce in weight, but somehow I cannot feel clean or correct at the table if my nails are black. Keep your nails short, use the brush with goop on it, and you'll be clean even following bike repairs.

14. Fingernail clipper (1)

F. Miscellaneous

1. Pocket knife (1) - for the reasons I gave in Part Two, my choice is the Buck Esquire Model 501. (3 ounces, 3" blade, $23)

2. Sheath knife (1) - as you can see in the drawing of my bike fully loaded for the road, I carry a sheath knife mounted on the left side of the head tube. The blade should be stainless steel and thesheath made of good leather. I affix the sheath to the head tube with two toeclip straps - they do a fine job of holding the blade in place and serve as replacements should my pedal straps break. My choice is the Buck Pathfinder Model 105. Its size is just right for the usual chores of camping and for personal protection. (7 ounces, 5" blade, $23)

3. Sunglasses with case (1)

4. Flashlight with batteries -I carry the Mallory Compact with two AA Duracell batteries. (3 ounces, $2.50)

5. Camera and film - the kind of camera you tour with, and the number of rolls of film you take along are so personal a choice that I won't suggest anything here aside from two packing and processing tips. First, make sure you keep your camera dry. This can be accomplished with any number of small, treated cordura or nylon bags, or the specially-made plastic Pocket Pouches and Phoenix Dry Bags. Next, do not pack your camera in the left side panniers, for this is the side you'll lay your bike on if your weight is such that a kickstand won't hold it up. Place it in the right side panniers, or in your handlebar bag if the zipper is easily accessible and the camera not so heavy that it throws off your steering. One final option - affix a water-proof camera bag to the rear of your saddle. I own a Yak Works catalogue bag called the Zoom Pak 35 ($30). It is padded, can be worn around the neck or strapped to a waist belt when off the bike, and is designed to hold a large 35mm camera and one lens up to 5" long. When hiking I carry my camera (Canon 35mm, 1.2 lens) and binoculars together in the bag.

On long tours I rid myself of the weight of exposed film by using Kodak Prepaid Processing Mailers. (REI, 36 exposure slide film, $4.13.) I always shoot slides, as it is less expensive and lends more easily to recapturing the feel of a tour when blown up on a screen, rather than a tiny print. Another company, Seattle Film Works, also provides this service of mailer-envelopes. Although I have had some difficulty with their film failing to advance in my camera (and failed to receive any reply when I wrote them and asked what the problem could be. I seem to be the only one of several people locally who use their film who is not fully satisfied. Seattle Film Works (address in appendix) uses plastic slide mounts, and provides a slide and negative, thus doing away with costly and quality-reducing interneg step when making enlargements from slides.

6. Rope (15' extremely thin braid, preferably parachute cord) -this is great for drying clothes at night, and as a good backup for a broken tent pole or lost shock cord. Check the surplus stores for parachute cord, or buy the 5 cent per foot cord from REI. Do not take clothesline.

7. Ripstop repair tape - 6", V2 ounce, 35 cents.

8. Matches -I carry one box of waterproof matches on tour (REI,

12 boxes for $1), but when these run out I pick up a book of matches in a cafe and keep them with my medical gear in a zip-lock bag.

9. Notebook - I carry the spiral stenographer's pad for journal notes and letters.

10. Book - paperback, not too heavy.

11. Ink pen (1)

12. Safety pins - the morning Wayne and I took off in '74 my grandfather handed me a small bag of pins and said he thought they'd come in handy. He was right, as usual, and ever since I've packed ten of different sizes in a film canister. They are great for quick repairs; a longer sewing job can thus be put off till evening in camp.

13. Sewing kit - one small needle, one large, and one spool of very heavy, tough thread are all I carry in this kit. The small needle does double duty in finding splinters, assisted by the tiny forceps on the Swiss Army Knife. (No. 0 Army suture if you can find it.)

14. Cup (1) -1 carry one metal cup (with handle) which is sufficient for making instant coffee, tea or soup over a campfire. Long ago I decided that carrying a stove was more trouble than it was worth, though you might choose to do so for long winter tours. Should you decide on a stove I suggest the one I've recently purchased as a replacement for my Optimus 8R - the Coleman Peak 1. Its considerable weight is offset by the features of a large fuel tank, extremely simple operation, and 8500 BTUH output (enough heat to boil a quart of water in 3 minutes).

Winter tours taken with a large group might take advantage of the reduced per-man weight and carry this stove, and the Coleman Peak 1 lantern. Also relatively light-weight, it would do much to extend the day past the 5:30 p.m. sundown which is a drawback of winter touring. And operated inside a tent, it will warm the air considerably. (Don't have the tent sealed up tight if the lantern is going, however.)

15. Utensil set - try the knife, fork and teaspoon made of Lexan (Early Winters, $1.80). They'll last a lifetime.

16. Can opener - GI type, REI, ½ ounce, 25 cents. Even though your Swiss Army Knife has an opener the GI type is worth the $1/_4$ ounce due to its speed and ease.

17. Panniers - see Part Two.

18. Plastic pannier covers - all good pannier material will retard water, but some is bound to make it inside. To keep your gear dry, you may inexpensively pack your belongings into individual plastic bags, or purchase specially made Eclipse pannier rain covers ($15, Bikecology). This latter method is much simpler, though considerably more expensive.

19. Pants clips

G. Tools

Most of this section will be a simple list of those items which I discussed in Part Two. Costs and locations can be found there.

1. crescent wrench - 6"
2. screwdriver - 6" overall length, regular blade
3. needle-nose pliers - smallest available with sidecutters
4. channel locks - 7"
5. tire levers (2)
6. allen wrenches - be sure you have a wrench for every allen head bolt or screw of different size on your bike.
7. cone wrenches (2)
8. chain rivet tool
9. spoke wrench ^-type*
10. freewheel tool
11. cotterless crank removal tool
12. Swiss Army Knife - Champion

H. Bike parts

1. brake cables (2)
2. gear cables (2)
3. brake pads (2)
4. ball bearings - replacement bearings for entire bike except for headset.
5. bearing grease - one tube Phil Wood
6. oil - small no-drip can, or better still a plastic bottle large enough to hold two or three ounces and equipped with a flip-lock top. I have purchased these small empty vials for 49 cents at drugstores.
7. chain links (5)
8. tube (1) - regular weight, not PR. This way, if a flat comes during the ride the good tube can be slapped in quickly, and the repair of the PR can be made at camp that night.
9. tire (1) - let me try to explain how you can fold a clincher tire and not damage the bead. First, holding the tire in front of you with your hands at the 3 and 9 o'clock positions, pull your hands together at your chest. (You now have two long oval loops which meet at your hand.) With your left hand take hold of both sides of the tire, thus freeing your right hand to reach through the lower loop, bending your arm upward to take hold of the upper loop. Now pull that loop toward you, still holding either side of the tire with your left hand. As you pull it closer you will notice that you have created two more loops in your tire; gradually release your left hand and these loops will fold upon themselves, resulting in a small, round, folded clincher with the metal bead intact.

Wayne and I learned this simple trick from a bike shop owner in England, who patiently stood by while we practiced the technique and told us of his days with Montgomery in North Africa. Not only were his stories fascinating, but by teaching us how to fold a tire he saved us from riding through the Middle East (where we had decided to pack two extra clinchers each) with tires strung around our necks like ammunition belts.

10. shock cords (2) - two cords beyond those required to hold your gear securely

11. spokes (6) - see Part Two on packing tips.

12. riding flag - a must.

13. fenders

14. air pump - Zefal high pressure.

15. air pressure gauge - Schraeder type for most, $3

16. luggage racks - front and rear (and make sure your mounting bolts tap into the frame eyelets for strength).

17. water bottles -1 ride with two in winter, three in summer.

18. reflectors - in rear of pedals, at end of rear rack. I try my best not to ride after dark on tour, and always remove my generator set from the bike because of the weight. But, if you are caught on the road at night your flashlight will give you some protection to the front, your reflectors to the rear.

19. lock and cable - Citadels are of course too heavy for touring. Also, you can't stray too far from your loaded bike for fear that your panniers will be stolen. Pack a thin cable and small key-padlock (make sure both of you have a key), and remember that this cable will serve only as a deterrent to someone jumping on your bike and pedalling off. One cable and lock per two riders; merely lock the two bikes together when in a cafe or at night in camp. When sightseeing I search out a fire station or friendly neighbor who will let me leave my bike in his care.

20. rear view mirror

21. toe clips and straps

22. tube repair kit -1 stuff the contents of two repair kits into one -two tubes of glue, and twice the original number of patches.

Final Checklist
A. Clothing
1. T-shirts (3)
2. long-sleeved shirt (1)
3. riding shorts (2)
4. belt(l)

5. undershorts (3)
6. long pants (1)
7. gym shorts (1)
8. insulated underwear (1 pair)
9. Protogs (1 pair leggings)
10. socks (3 pairs)
11. riding shoes (1 pair)
12. camp moccasins (1 pair)
13. bandanas(2)
14. riding gloves (1 pair)
15. baseball cap (1)

B. Foul and cold weather gear
1. boots (1 pair)
2. neck gaiter (1)
3. wool cap (1)
4. jacket (1)
5. gloves (1 pair)
6. poncho (1)
7. rain chaps (1 pair)
8. rain suit (1)
9. rain cap (1)
10. rain boots (1 pair)
11. goggles (1)
12. down or fiberfill jacket (1)

C. Shelter and bedding
1. tent(l)
2. sleeping bag (1)
3. ground pad (1)

D. Medical supplies
1. sunshade (1 bottle)
2. aspirin (20)
3. snakebite kit (1)
4. Desitin (1 tube)
5. hydrogen peroxide (1 bottle)
6. band-aids (10)
7. butterfly closure bandages (6)
8. combat bandage (1)
9. gauze compress pads (4- 8)
10. gauze (1 roll)

11. ace bandage (1)
12. petroleum jelly (1 tube)
13. Benadryl (1 bottle)
14. insect repellent (1 bottle)
15. water purification tablets (1 bottle)
16. moleskin (1 pad)

E. Personal

1. towel (1)
2. washcloth (1)
3. soap (1)
4. soapdish (1)
5. toothbrush (1)
6. toothbrush case (1)
7. tooth powder (I bottle)
8. comb (1)
9. toilet paper (20 sheets)
10. deodorant (1)
11. shampoo (I bottle)
12. waterless hand cleaner (1 tube)
13. nail brush (1)
14. fingernail clipper (1)

F. Miscellaneous

1. pocket knife (1)
2. sheath knife (1)
3. sunglasses/case (1)
4. flashlight/batteries (1)
5. camera/film (1)
6. rope (15')
7. ripstop repair tape (6")
8. matches (1 box)
9. notebook (1)
10. book (1)
11. pen(l)
12. safety pins (10)
13. sewing kit (1)
14. cup (1)
15. utensil set (1)
16. can opener (1)
17. panniers (I set)
18. plastic pannier covers (1 set)

19. pants clips (2)

G. *Tools*
1. crescent wrench (1)
2. screwdriver (1)
3. needle-nose pliers (1)
4. channel locks (1)
5. tire levers (2)
6. allen wrenches
7. cone wrenches (2)
8. chain rivet tool (1)
9. spoke wrench (1)
10. freewheel tool (1)
11. cotterless crank removal tool (1)
12. Swiss Army Knife (1)

H. *Bike parts*
1. brake cables (2)
2. gear cables (2)
3. brake pads (2)
4. ball bearings
5. bearing grease (1 tube)
6. oil(1 bottle)
7. chain links (5)
8. tube (1)
9. tire (1)
10. shock cords (2)
11. spokes (6)
12. riding flag (1)
13. fenders
14. air pump (1)
15. air gauge (1)
16. luggage racks (2)
17. water bottles (2 - 3)
18. reflectors
19. lock and cable *(1)*
20. rear view mirror (1)
21. toe clips and straps (1 pair)
22. tube repair kit (1)

8. Packing and Riding the Touring Bike

The impressive list of touring equipment on the last few pages has no doubt caused you to wonder if you'll have room in your panniers for everything, and if you'll be able to pedal up hills with all the weight. Well. Don't worry. It will be a tight fit to pack it all in, and it will take time to accustom yourself to riding with a full load, but you can do it. My tips on packing will deal primarily with weight distribution, as personal preference will ultimately decide the location of most items. And any guidance I can provide in riding a loaded bike is probably similar to what you might think to tell a child who is learning to ride for the first time - the words make sense to you because you already know how to do it, but very little to the kid until he has actually mounted up and fallen a few times. Therefore, please don't think I'm shortchanging you in these areas when I say very little about them;

The truth of the matter is that you'll gain more through your own experimentation in packing and riding that I can give you in a book.

If you flip back to the exercise chart you'll see that five of the twelve weeks are used in becoming accustomed to riding with weight. Week Eight begins with one-half of the expected tour weight; this is repeated in Week Nine, and then the other half is added for the final three weeks of training. I suggest this gradual escalation to prevent the shock which is present when a rider goes from a light-weight commuter's bag one day, to a full thirty pound touring set-up the next. Do this and you'll feel like you're trying to steer a truck. You'll be out of balance around curves, and you'll misjudge stopping distances, and you'll begin considering alternative vacations.

The two most common problems in packing seem to be:

a. putting so much weight in the handlebar bag that the front end steering is thrown out of true.

b. putting almost all the weight on the rear rack and thereby causing a 'mushy' feeling in the rear tire - a result of bowed spokes and a flattened out clincher.

Some riders suggest 60% of tour weight on the rear rack, 40% up front, but this can be only the crudest of guidelines. Let me try to be more helpful by telling you specifically where my major weight items are carried. You can try this first, and begin your own rearranging from there.

Weight is carried most easily on two wheels when kept low to the ground and close to the frame. Thus, I tour with front and rear panniers, as well as a handlebar bag. Almost two-thirds of my entire load is carried in the rear, but of the weight in front only a very small percentage is in the handlebar bag. This is due to the effect upon my steering which even the weight of my 35mm camera and one extra lens has when carried this high. Yet many times this weight can be packed in the front panniers without any appreciable effort. Therefore, in my handlebar bag I carry light-weight items which must be easily accessible - medical supplies, toothbrush and powder, sunglasses, film, flashlight, matches, utensils, maps. In the front panniers I carry rainwear, approximately one-half of my clothing, the camera and second lens. On the front rack, lying flat, is my folded clincher, with the down jacket (inside a waterproof stuff sack) lashed on top of it.

The tent, sleeping bag, and ground pad ride on the rear rack, mounted in such a way that their length is perpendicular to the rack. You might at first think this would create more wind resistance, but actually the bags do not extend more than an inch or so beyond my thighs on either side. The tent lies closest to the center of the bike, for as the heaviest item it would place undue stress upon the rear wheel were it mounted toward the back on the rear rack. The sleeping bag lies behind the tent, and the ground pad on top between the two.

Naturally, all your remaining gear will be located in your rear panniers. You must try your best to balance these bags in weight, and not to unthinkingly alter this balance by tossing all your newly purchased foodstuff into one pannier, or failing to replace an item in its original location. As soon as you find the best spot for each bit of gear (and this will take the entire training period and probably a week of actual riding on tour), make a list of each item's location in your journal " It will be an invaluable packing tip for the next ride. Also, if you keep things in the same pannier for all rides you'll soon know exactly where to find that one item you want, without looking through all your bags.

Most of you will probably tour with your spouse or a friend, in which case your per-bike load will be drastically reduced. For example, one set of tools is sufficient if you intend to ride together, or at least within eyesight of one another. If your practice rides have shown that your cyclic rates (pedal revolutions per minute) are greatly different and that several miles distance exists between you at all times, make sure the slower rider carries the tools. If he breaks down he can fix his bike and catch up; if the faster rider has a flat he merely waits for his buddy to arrive.

The best trade-off for one rider packing the tools is for the second rider to carry the tent. After this major exchange comes the following breakdown of gear. I have listed only those items which I find no reason to carry two of on tour, except as indicated below.

Slower rider
tools
all medical supplies
chain links
air gauge
air pump
Faster rider

tent
ball bearings
bearing grease
oil
lock/cable
flashlight/batteries
rope
ripstop repair tape
safety pins
sewing kit
can opener
fingernail clipper
nail brush
waterless hand cleaner
soap/soap dish
deodorant
shampoo
Note: the faster rider must

pack his own snakebite kit, combat bandage or compress pads and gauze roll, and Benadryl. Also the slower rider need not carry the ball bearings because bearing replacement is not an emergency-type repair.

One final item which is often shared by two riders is the camera, due to its considerable weight. However, to avoid later contention, decide *before* the ride whose camera will be used, who will purchase the film and keep the original slides or negatives, how the repair bill will be apportioned if something goes wrong, and how the replacement cost will be decided if the camera is lost or stolen.

Earlier I warned that you should gradually increase your bike load until it reaches full tour weight. I suggest the following method in doing this.

Begin by strapping your tent to the rear rack, your sleeping bag to the front rack. This will provide you with approximately nine pounds, or roughly one half the tour weight if you are riding with a partner of equal strength who will carry his share of the load. If you have been riding with a handlebar bag, the addition of the sleeping bag to the front rack will not greatly affect your steering. However, if this is the first time you'll have weight up front, then expect 'sluggish' steering.

The two most common remarks heard following a cyclist's first ride with weight have to do with decreased maneuverability and increased distance necessary to stop. Take some time to accustom yourself to these changes with half the tour weight, and then add partially filled rear panniers. (If they do not have the 'cut-away' design, you may have to position them more than once to keep your heels from hitting them on each pedal upstroke.) Next, remove the sleeping bag from up front and strap it into place behind the tent; attach your front panniers and add the handlebar bag. Again, each cyclist must learn his own weight limitation for this last bag, but do begin with light items. You should be able to lift your hands from the brake hoods while riding and feel your bike maintain its balance. If it instead veers sharply to one side, you should check the weight in your handlebar bag, or balance your right and left pannier loads in front and rear.

Finally, remember that the back of your bike is, when touring, as wide as your handlebars. Cyclists who have pedalled many miles together develop a 'lock-in' position on the road - not exactly riding double, but with the front tire of rider in back just to the left of the faster rider's rear tire. In this position they can talk to one another easily, and yet disengage quickly when a car appears; the man in rear merely stops pedalling, the front rider continues at normal speed, a distance of a few inches appears in only seconds and the rider in rear tucks himself nearly into single file. However, a handlebar bag and front panniers obscure a cyclist's view of his own front tire, and he must re-determine how close he can 'lock-in'.

Take your time becoming accustomed to touring weight, and don't forget that although you may be covering fewer miles at greater effort you are packing your shelter and repair shed with you. As you'll begin to understand when you pedal across states requesting only directions and buying food, there's much to be said for being self-contained.

9. Life on the Road

In this final section I want to offer a few observations which might make touring more interesting, and perhaps a bit easier for you. You are, by now, knowledgeable of the bike and general touring equipment which you will require for life on the road. But, until you actually begin cycling cross-country you might find it difficult to imagine how truly different travelling by bicycle is from racing about in a car. Naturally, you'll be planning your first tour before you have this experience, and therefore these final words.

Make your first tour an easy one.. By this I refer to daily mileages in the 35 to 50 range, and less if in rough terrain. When motorists plan a vacation it generally involves a destination many hundreds of miles distant; the country between home and the intended vacation spot is to be covered as quickly, and therefore as painlessly, as possible. Often a family will leave late at night or long before dawn to avoid traffic on the highways. Gratification during these travel times may come in part from the scenery, but mostly from the steady ticking off of miles on the odometer. Stops are limited both in number and duration, and the unrelieved boredom of hours behind the wheel is offset by the knowledge that if a certain speed is maintained, the destination will be reached a half-hour earlier than planned. In short, the vacation begins Just as the normal workday - in your car, concerned with traffic, and worrying about making good time.

With this background of experience how is the motorist-turned-biker likely to plan his tour? Chances are he'll choose a destination an impressive distance from his home, one requiring far more hours in the saddle than he might like once he begins. Having spent a lifetime gauging progress on the road by miles travelled, he is now likely to experience dissatisfaction with the comparatively paltry distance he can pedal. Obviously, a biker cannot think like a motorist and enjoy his ride. But you would be surprised at the number of cyclists who unknowingly try to do Just that.

To break these motorist habits you must first decide that your destination is merely a turn-around or stopping point, and not the totality of your tour. You will be travelling at a speed much more human than that allowed cars, and likewise your thoughts should leave the technology of time and speed computations, to focus on nature and man. Leave your wristwatch at home, awaken when you're rested, eat when you are hungry, and sleep when you are tired. Such natural actions, and simple thoughts, are a true vacation from the modern world.

Many days I have watched the sun come up over my front tire and set over my rear, creating shadows of various lengths through the day as my bike and I served as a giant sundial. Watching these shadows gives a different perception of time than that cold number blinking out from a digital watch. What cycle touring does in this regard is to destroy that terrible invention of the early nineteenth century, that necessary coordinate of industrialization - disciplined time.

It may sound silly that modern man has little time to think, especially given the greater number of leisure hours which we enjoy. Yet we organize these free hours, as though afraid to give our mind free rein. Touring forces that freedom upon us; that opportunity to think creatively. I will wager that almost every one of you, after a week's touring, will be either extremely bored with the time you have in the saddle, or be fascinated with the directions your mind will take when given the hours to think. I have yet to find someone in the middle of these two positions.

For instance, I recall a weekend ride when in high school, with some friends from a science class. We had been studying astronomy, and one of the most interesting questions to arise concerned the number of directions the earth moved at the same time. We all knew it rotated on its axis, that it revolved around the sun, that the galaxy moved through space. Somehow on that ride I focused upon the similarity of the ball bearings in a pedal; they rotate within their bearing cups, revolve around the pedal axle, spin in a circle about the crank, travel

a linear path down the road, rotate with the earth, revolve around the
. . . and so it went, on and on in my mind. Suddenly, what had been
some stranger's concept became for me creative thought, and did so
only when I had time to think.

Now, I suppose a genius could sit in a room and keep himself
company forever. And on the other end exist those poor folk who must
always have a television or radio nearby. My own weak brain falls in
between, as most do, and cycling fits these perfectly. The stimula-
tion of the morning paper at breakfast in a cafe, a day of small towns
and natural sights broken up by hours in the saddle alone with my
thoughts or sharing them with a friend - this is the best combination
for me. There's time to learn the crops by sight, to predict the weather
by clouds overhead, to wonder at the dreams and despair which might
make up the story of abandoned farmhouses and businesses along the
trail. All this is yours if you can break the habits of being in a hurry.

Deal with transportation problems before the tour. The easiest
tour to plan is a round-trip from your home, but if you must travel
somewhere to begin the journey I strongly suggest that you gather
all the necessary information on shipping your bike before the trip
begins. This is due to the special requirements for travelling with a
bike by bus, rail, or plane. For instance, Amtrak provides a bicycle
box for $4, but requests a three day notice prior to your departure
date. There is no additional fee for handling, as the bike will count
as one of the three pieces of luggage you are allowed. However, you
must ask if a baggage car will be attached to your train; otherwise
your bike remains behind. (Bike boxes require the removal of pedal
and turning of handlebars. I use all the space in the box by cramming
my panniers, tent and sleeping bag inside.)

Greyhound and Continental Trailways also allow a bike to be
checked as one piece of luggage, but cannot guarantee that your
bike will arrive at its destination on the same bus you do - it depends
upon available space. These buslines do not provide boxes, so you will
have to obtain them from bike shops in your town. Ask long before
your tour, as most shops destroy their boxes once they're empty. (I've
never had to pay for a box from a bike shop, but don't balk at some
nominal fee.) Continental Trailways places a minimum size limitation
upon boxes - 8" x32" x60".

The airlines change their policies periodically, so you should
contact them before you arrive at the airport. Several now provide
a one-time fee of $14 for a box and transportations costs, though
occasionally a carrier will still accept an unboxed bike. Actually,
this is a safer method of travel, for the handlers load the bike in last
and set nothing on top of it; in a box the bike gets tossed about and

often winds up under other luggage. In the past I've had no trouble on international flights by putting my heavy tools and camera in the handlebar bag and claiming this as carry-on baggage, with the result that the bike box weighed close to the thirty-two or so pound limitation. But a work of caution - some airlines have unpressurized baggage compartments which might cause your tires to blow. Always reduce your air pressure by half when flying, or ask the agent about this when purchasing your ticket.

Dealing with all these questions beforehand will assure you an untroubled journey, and keep you from becoming separated from your bike. Until travel with bicycles becomes commonplace, a single policy will not be hammered out; check for changes from year to year even when riding with the same rail, bus or airline.

Don't think the only place to camp is a campground. Farmers are usually hospitable to small groups of cyclists who ask only to borrow a few tent-sized patches of earth for one night; jails will sometimes put you up, churches in small towns will often open up a basement or let you camp on a lawn. Small town city parks are generally off-limits to camping, and are noisy, busy spots anyway. But if there is nowhere else to stay, a request to a sheriff might be successful. Don't expect to be welcomed if a campground is just a few miles down the road, or if an inexpensive motel is nearby. But if such facilities are far away most people will be helpful, if you are travelling the backroads. Towns, and the people in them, seem to take on a different attitude when major highways run down Main Street. Perhaps it is an understandable decrease in trust, or an equally unfortunate acquisitive spirit. Whatever the reason you should avoid major highways whenever possible.

Be thoughtful in traffic. By this I mean not only to be careful, but to be aware of the motorists' feelings as well as your own. Countless passing cars will honk to say hello, never suspecting that they have disturbed a peaceful thought or almost scared you off your saddle. The driver or passenger will wave, and responding amiably becomes a chore. But at least nod your head and smile, for many times I have met these people down the road where they have stopped to eat or spend the night, and would have felt ill at ease had I been sullen when they honked.

A second group of drivers to be thoughtful of on the road are truckers. The popular conception of these men as cowboys out for fun tends to impart in a cyclist's mind immediate malevolent intent when a truck passes fast and close. I have met up with truck drivers who I thought had risked my life for grins, and confronted them about it.

Without exception their replies have shown me how quickly a cyclist can do that which we accuse motorists of constantly - thinking only of themselves on the road. The truckers have explained that whereas I take up only three feet of space, their rigs require an entire lane, and that on a two-lane road without a shoulder this puts them well across the center line if they pass me with even a three foot berth. Further enlightenment along the lines of a need to keep up the rpm (revolutions per minute) of their engine so as to make it up a hill, or the noise of air brakes not being intended to scare a rider off the road, has helped me to give the close-passing truck the benefit of the doubt. And doing so makes for a happier ride.

Well. I guess that's about it. I have a hundred commuting and touring stories I'd like to tell, but in the time you're reading mine you could be on the road gathering your own. And that is, after all, what this book has been about getting you on two wheels. So have fun, and be careful. And wave as you pedal by.

Appendices

$$\text{inch gear} \quad = \quad \frac{\text{\#teeth front sprocket}}{\text{\#teeth rear sprocket}} \text{ x wheel diameter in inches}$$

for example: $\dfrac{54}{14} \text{ x } 27 = 104 \text{ inch gear}$

Gear Chart for 27" Wheel

Number of teeth in front sprocket

	24	26	28	30	32	34	36	38	40	42	44	45	46	47	48	49	50	52	53	54	55	56
12	54	58.5	63	67.5	72	76.5	81	85.5	90	94.5	99	101.2	103.5	105.7	108	110.2	112.3	117	119.3	121.5	122.7	126
13	49.8	54	58.1	62.6	66.4	70.8	74.7	78.9	83.1	87	91.4	93.4	95.5	97.6	99.7	101.8	103.9	108	110	112.1	114.2	116.3
14	46.2	50.1	54	57.8	61.7	65.5	69.5	73.3	77.1	81.2	84.9	86.7	88.7	90.6	92.6	94.5	96.4	100.3	102.2	104.1	106	108
15	43.2	46.8	50.4	54	57.6	61.1	64.8	68.4	72.	75.6	79.2	81	82.8	84.6	86.4	88.2	90	93.6	95.4	97.2	99	100.8
16	40.5	43.7	47.2	50.6	54	57.2	60.9	64.1	67.5	70.9	74.3	76	77.6	79.3	81	82.7	84.4	87.8	89.4	91.1	92.8	94.5
17	38.1	41.2	44.4	47.6	50.8	54	57.2	60.3	63.5	66.7	69.9	71.5	73.1	74.6	76.2	77.8	79.4	82.6	84.1	85.7	87.3	88.9
18	36	39	42	45	48	51	54	57	60	63	66	67.5	69	70.5	72	73.5	75	78	79.5	81	82.5	84
19	34.1	36.8	39.7	42.6	45.5	48.2	51.1	54	56.8	59.7	62.5	64	65.4	66.8	68.2	69.6	71.1	73.9	75.3	76.7	78.1	79.5
20	32.4	35.1	37.8	40.5	43.2	45.9	48.7	51.3	54	4637	59.4	60.8	62.1	63.4	64.8	662	67.5	70.2	71.5	72.9	74.5	75.6
21	30.8	33.4	36	38.6	41.1	43.7	46.4	48.9	51.4	54	56.6	57.9	59.1	60.4	61.7	63	64.3	6639	68.1	69.4	70.7	72
22	29.4	31.9	34.3	36.8	3902	41.6	44.2	46.6	49.1	51.5	54	55.2	56.5	57.6	58.9	60.1	61.4	63.8	65	66.2	67.5	68.7
23	28.1	30.5	32.8	35.2	37.5	39.9	42.4	46.6	47	49.3	51.6	52.8	54	55.2	56.3	57.5	58.7	61	62.2	63.6	64.5	65.7
24	27	29.2	31.5	33.7	36	38.2	40.5	42.8	45	47.3	49.5	50.7	51.8	52.9	54	55.1	56.3	58.6	59.6	60.7	61.8	63
25	25.9	28	30.2	32.4	34.6	36.7	38.9	41	43.2	45.4	47.5	48.6	49.7	50.8	51.8	52.9	54	56.2	57.2	58.3	59.4	60.4
26	24.9	27	29	31.2	33.2	35.3	37.4	39.5	41.5	4.3.6	45.7	46.7	47.8	48.8	49.9	50.9	51.9	54	55	56	57.1	58.1
28	23.1	25	27	28.9	30.8	32.8	32.8	36.6	38.6	40.5	42.4	43.4	44.4	45.3	46.3	47.2	48.2	50.1	51.1	52	53	54
29	22.4	24.2	26.1	28	29.8	31.6	33.5	35.4	37.2	39	41	41.9	42	43.8	44.7	45.6	46.5	48.4	49.4	50.3	51.2	52.1
30	21.6	23.4	25.2	27	28.8	30.6	324	34.2	36	37.8	39.6	40.5	41.4	42.3	43.2	44.1	45	46.8	47.7	48.6	49.5	50.4
31	20.9	22.6	24.4	26.2	27.9	29.6	31.4	33.1	34.8	36.6	38.3	39.2	40.1	41	41.8	42.6	43.5	45.2	46.2	47	47.9	48.8
32	20.3	22	23.6	25.3	27	28.7	30.4	32.1	33.7	35.4	37.2	38	38.8	39.7	40.5	41.4	42.2	43.9	44.7	45.5	46.4	47.3
33	19.6	21.3	22.9	24.6	26.2	27.8	29.5	31.1	32.7	34.4	36	36.8	37.6	38.5	39.3	40.1	40.9	42.6	43.4	44.2	45	45.9
34	19.1	20.6	22.2	23.8	25.4	27	28.6	30.2	31.8	33.3	35	35.7	36.5	37.4	38.1	38.9	39.7	41.3	42.1	42.9	43.6	44.5

Number of teeth in rear sprocket

Bicycle Catalogues and Accessories

Mail Order:

Bikecology
4051 Lincoln Blvd
Marina Del Rey, CA 90292
Call us: 310-821-0766
Email us: Info@Bikecology-MDR.com
Web: http://www.bikecolo-gymdr.com

Lickton's Cycle City
310 Lake St.
Oak Park, 111. 60302
(708) 383-2130
http://www.lickbike.com/

Palo Alto Bicycles
171 University Ave
Palo Alto, CA 94301
(650) 328-7411
http://www.paloaltobicycles.com/

Bike Nashbar
Nashbar
6103 St Rt 446
Canfield, Ohio
United States 44406
1-877-688-8600

http://www.nashbar.com

Burley Design
4685 Cloudburst Way
Eugene, OR 97402
Tel: 541-687-1644
Toll Free (US & Canada): 800-311-5294
Fax: 541-687-0436
Email: burley@burley.com
http://www.burley.com

Accessories:

Bell Helmets, Inc.
Helmet Support
949 Newhall St.
1-800-341-5834
(949) 574-2890
Costa Mesa, Ca. 92627
support@bellhelmets.com
http://www.bellhelmets.com/

AVOCET Incorporated
180 Constitution Dr.#2
Menlo Park, CA. 94025
Tel. 650-470-0478
Fax. 650-470-0490

http://www.avocet.com/

byKart
P.O. Box 8373
Fountain Valley, CA 92708

Troxel Manufacturing Co.
Highway 57
Moscow, Tenn. 38057
Tel 901.877.6875
http://www.troxel.com/
info@troxel.com

Organizations:
American Youth Hostels

891 Amsterdam Avenue
New York, NY 10025-4403
Phone: (212) 932-2300
http://www.hiusa.org/

League of American Wheelmen
1612 K Street NW, Suite 800
Washington, DC 20006-2850
Phone: (202) 822-1333
Fax: (202) 822-1334
Email: bikeleague@bikeleague.org
http://www.bikeleague.org

Magazines:
Bicycling Magazine
33 E. Minor
St. Emmaus, PA 18049
http://www.bicycling.com/
Tel (800)-666-2806
Trailspace
P.O. Box 499
Belgrade Lakes, ME 04918-0499 USA

feedback@trailspace.com
http://www.trailspace.com/

Panniers:
Lone Peak Panniers
3474 South 2300 East
Salt Lake City, Utah 84109
Tel 800.777.7679
http://www.lonepeakpacks.com/

The Touring Cyclist
11816 Saint Charles Rock Rd
Bridgeton, MO
63044-2610
314.739.4648
314.739.5183

Cannondale Corporation
35 Pulaske Street
Stamford, Connecticut 06902
USA: 1-800-726-2453
http://www.cannondalestation.com

Appendix C

General Outdoor Distributors

Recreational Equipment Inc. (REI)
Sumner, WA 98352-0001
800-426-4840
http://www.rei.com/

Eastern Mountain Sports (EMS)
Vose Farm Road
Peterborough, NH 03458
888-463-6367
http://www.ems.com/home/
index.jsp

Sierra Designs
Sierra Designs Headquarters
6235 Lookout Road, Suite C
Boulder, CO 80301
http://www.sierradesigns.com/
800.736.8592

Sahalie (Formerly Early Winters, Ltd.)
3188 NW Aloclek Drive
Hillsboro, OR 97124
1-800-458-4438
http://www.sahalie.com/

L.L. Bean, Inc.
Freeport, Maine 04033
800-441-5713
http://www.llbean.com/

North Face
The North Face®
14450 Doolittle Drive
San Leandro, CA 94577 USA
1-866-715-3223
http://www.thenorthface.com

The Ski Hut
1032 East 4th Street
Duluth, MN
218.724.8525
http://www.theskihut.com

PEAK 1 (lanterns)
The Coleman Company, Inc.
3600 N Hydraulic St,
Wichita, KS 67201
316.832.2653
800.835.3278
http://www.coleman.com/

The Rivendell Mountain works
PO BOX 622,
Monroe, WA. 98272
Phone 425-788-7892 (evenings only, or leave message)
http://rivendellmountainworks.
com